CREATIVE MIND

CREATIVE MIND

A Diary of Teenage Mental Illness

Nicole Nagy

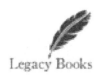

Legacy Books

Creative Mind: A Diary of Teenage Mental Illness
First Edition

Copyright © 2017 by Nicole Nagy

Published in the United States of America by Legacy Books

For more information, please contact the author at
acreativemind.tdotmi@gmail.com

ISBN - 13: 978-1979500555
ISBN - 10: 197950055X

Edited by David Tabatsky
Cover and interior design by Jill M. Pozderec

For anyone struggling with mental illness

September 25, 2009

I want to drop out of school and go somewhere far away. I cry some nights, locked in my room, squirming, rolling around in my bed, fighting to get the words out.

"Mom."

Nothing.

"Dad."

Nope.

My body is stuck. My mind is processing the words, but my mouth is not opening. I lay there, defenseless.

I can't defend myself against myself!

Finally, I calm down enough to leave my room and approach my mom, who asks me a familiar question without much emotion—maybe that's 'cause she asks it every day.

"Nicole, is everything okay?"

Nothing comes out. All I want is to be held by my mom and for her to tell me everything is going to be okay. Although in my mind, it was clear that it was *not* going to be okay and these episodes are going to continue and I can't stop them.

At school, I feel out of place, like I am some kind of altered version of a human being.

What's my purpose of living?

I ask myself that all the time.

Why should I live?

I ask myself that and don't have much of an answer.

I'm crap and nobody likes me anyway.

My mind tells me that when I hear voices in my head. I know they are not real, but they are real enough for me. I hear the usual things.

I'm a piece of shit.

When I hear stuff like this enough inside my head I come to the conclusion that these voices are right and I can't win this argument with myself.

Whenever I'm at school I feel so scared that I might say the wrong thing or something that will not come out just right or it will be too fast or too slow. Then I feel forced to over explain myself or apologize. Sometimes I get angry because I feel like I don't understand people. Or they don't understand me, which is probably happening all the time.

I just shrug it off and say things to myself.

Ah well, I'll be gone by tomorrow.

I don't even know where I will be gone to, or what I mean when I say that, or maybe I do, and it's really weird shit I'm thinking, and I shouldn't be, but I can't help it.

Will I be gone by tomorrow, or some other day?

Why am I even asking this? Is it because I don't want to be where I am? Does that mean in school, or home, in my room—or maybe it means in my life, like I won't stay in my life tomorrow?

Maybe these are the meds I'm taking, talking to me, which is why I can't figure anything out about myself, because my brain is all messed up.

Is it?

There must be some explanation.

What is wrong with me?

Author's Note

This episode may sound somewhat familiar to some people, but I know I was not the average teenager, in spite of trying so hard to be one. That's because I was grappling with mental illness, which affected most every part of my daily existence for many years.

This is the story of my life—how I first encountered mental illness, which led to a seizure condition and brain surgery, and how I learned to navigate my way to success as a young woman.

Although I may be controversial in this book here and there, my memory can be a little foggy, so if I say something more than once or twice, I apologize.

The language in the book is somewhat strong at times but it does not reflect the way I generally speak out loud. Anxiety and depression can trigger strong emotional reactions and extreme thinking, and a creative mind often tends to amplify those feelings.

Then again, from an early age—according to my mom—I had allergies and ear infections and terrible coughing fits and I couldn't sit still and I threw stuff at my speech therapist and then got diagnosed with something that turned out years later to be wrong.

I will stop here and let my journal entries and memories speak for themselves, as I try to unwind the path that lead to where I am today in the hopes that we can all come to a better understanding of how the brain works and how challenging it can be for so many kids grappling in the shadows with these issues.

September 4, 2008

Today was the last day of summer and tomorrow is my first day of freshman year at Sachem North High School. What kind of name is that? The school is located in Lake Ronkonkoma, which means my mom has to drive me to school because it's very far away.

I'm not going to lie. I'm terrified out of my mind. It's getting later and later into the night and I am freaking out. I think I sinned more than enough times for me to not make it into heaven.

Please let me fucking die.

Please let some terrible shit happen to me.

That's what I am thinking, and I'm swearing out of my mind right now, wishing all kinds of bad things to happen to me, like getting hit by a car within the next few hours, or like by chance if I was emptying the garbage and something big fell on my head, or I could have a brain aneurysm, or die of natural causes in my sleep, like my heart would just stop or something like that—nothing too gory, obviously.

My parents tried to calm me down. My grandmother is unaware of what's going on. I dread going to school tomorrow and all I can keep doing is telling God to take me already so I won't have to go to school.

This all started last month when my family and I moved to Kings Park, New York from the Poconos in Pennsylvania. Three previous deals on a new house didn't go through because of all different kinds of stuff I don't fully understand, but it sucks. My family and I had no choice but to move into my grandmother's home here on Long Island until we can find a house because I have to start high school.

My childhood growing up was pretty normal, except I did notice that I was brought to more doctors than my sister, Alisa, who is four years older than me. I thought it was normal, always seeing different specialists and taking dozens of different medications for allergies and coughing all the time and ADD and headaches, and this one episode I had, which I remember so vividly. I was six or seven years old when I experienced a very strong tantrum. I was lying on the green carpet of our living room in our house on Eastern Long Island, on a hot summer day, trying to control every force in my body while my mom was on the phone with my doctor.

"You have to help her," she said on the speaker phone. "This medication is messing with her—she is not herself!"

I tried with all of my might, squirming on the carpet, to hold in my screams, but I was unsuccessful because I kept screaming at the top of my lungs.

Could this have been the start of my seizures at such a young age?

According to my mother, I was restless pretty much from birth, which was originally attributed possibly to an allergy to almost any baby formula. My mom took me constantly to the pediatrician for ear infections. Then, when I was two, I got a chronic cough at night and then I had difficulty speaking and my words seemed muffled. The pediatrician checked my hearing and I had to go to the doctor over and over to see if I had fluid in my ears. I guess I had speech difficulty at the age of two and did speech therapy, and my mom says I rarely listened to the speech teacher and threw my toys at her. Yikes! I hope I didn't hurt her! I guess I couldn't sit still for even a few minutes at a time. Eventually, my speech improved and when I was three I supposedly was advanced for my age when it came to expressive speech.

When my mother took me to a reading group at the local library I was always fighting and wanting to leave and at home I was always very active running up and down the stairs as fast as I could. There was no way I would sit down and do anything. I started kindergarten when I was four years old and ten months and it was hard for me because I had trouble focusing and sitting still.

My teacher suggested I get checked for a condition called ADHD and when they evaluated me I was diagnosed with ADD, but they didn't put me on any meds. They just said I should be in a smaller class with less children so I could get more attention and stuff. My father took me to doctors all the time for earaches, stomachaches, and headaches. This continued all through first grade, and when I was six I started coughing every night and this lasted for a few years so I had to have this nebulizer treatment.

I was not able to concentrate in grade school, which always led teachers to treat me differently, and I was even held back a year in school. Other than that, I've lived a pretty normal life, with two loving parents and my sister is cool, even though during our childhood she thought I was a real piece of work. My mom was a nurse and my dad worked with computers.

I've always heard people say that the adolescent years are the most challenging. Boy, they weren't kidding! I've never been nervous going to school before. I always enjoyed it, even when I didn't do very well. But high school is a different story because it's such a new, really big change—for me, and for everybody starting high school.

I don't know anybody and it's not like I will have any of my friends from middle school to help me. All my friends are in a different state! At least everyone else has a buddy or friend of some kind they can stick with, but not me because so far I am all on my own.

September 5, 2008

My mom drove me to school. We arrived at 7:10 a.m. I sat in the car, looking at my mom.

"Are you sure you want to do this" I said to her, as if she had a gun and was about to pull the trigger.

She laughed.

"You'll be fine."

I was glued to my seat with no desire to take off my seatbelt. All I wanted was to hide.

Who needs school?

My mom tried to calm me with positive thoughts.

"You're going to do great"!

I was getting rushing thoughts in my head, like "You're right, easy for you to say," and "Yep, I'm going to be shoved into a locker today by a big kid!"

When it was time for me to go I thought I was going to die of fear right there on the spot. I got out of the car somehow and went around to give my mom a hug, hoping for more words of encouragement, which she had, for sure, but by the time I approached the front door of the school they were not helping.

I entered the building and pulled out my schedule.

F110, Earth Science.

I started walking, even though I had no idea where this class was or where the hallway was leading. I kept my head down, petrified that I might break down and collapse into a fetal position. When I found an assistant principal's office, I ran inside, out of breath. Maybe I was hyperventilating from stress.

I asked the lady at the front desk to show me where my class was and she helped me. I found it creepy and comforting that she could tell how nervous I was.

How did I give that away?

I can't stop thinking this.

The classroom was small with maybe ten or 11 students. The kids stared at me, which made me want to throw up. I couldn't help it. I put my head down and just prayed to God that something would happen so I could go home. The class started and I kept quiet, trying not to draw any attention to myself.

I got lucky when there was a knock on the door and it was for me. It was a teacher who I later found out was my guidance counselor. Her name was Ms. Roell and she was positively the nicest women I ever met.

I walked with her down to her office. I asked if I was in trouble and she laughed and shook her head. She went over my class schedule, explained some rules, and introduced me to one of the social workers, Ms. Samrouski, but I call her Ms. S. for short because it's obviously easier to remember. I went down to her office and she went over my file, too, and said my mom called, saying I should talk to her.

What the heck is a social worker, anyway?

I guess that means she talks a lot. Ms. S. asked me questions about what I enjoyed doing. She was basically trying to determine how sad my life was, like did I have any friends? What did I like to do for fun? Do I have any fun? Am I able to make friends easily? What are my needs? Am I secretly a serial killer? Normal stuff!

She said I would be visiting her once or twice a week to talk and catch up and that I would really like the school staff because they were helpful and supportive. She told me if I needed anything I could ask, which made me remember the hallway situation, which I couldn't stop thinking about since I entered school in the morning.

"Can I leave early from class?" I said, hoping that being so brutally honest wouldn't get me in trouble. "Because I'm terrified to walk the halls by myself when the bell rings."

I already had a plan to take advantage of this every

chance I got because I felt like a little fish swimming in a pool with giant sharks. Everybody else was bigger than me. Kids who were seniors looked like they were college students, and everybody was loud.

October 5, 2008

I decided to try out for the school soccer team. I played soccer all my life and even though I was scared my family encouraged me to do it because it would help me meet people. Another thing I was scared of was change, because it meant new people and I would have to explain myself all over again.

It's always the same questions.

Where are you from?

Huh, where is that?

What's your name?

Whatever.

I found the other girls to be freakishly huge like they were all on steroids. I didn't expect tryouts to be easy, but I guess I was a little off my game since I hadn't played in a couple of months since we moved. I felt I was being picked on and getting beat up, but I guess everybody feels that way, especially if you're a freshman.

I have a lot of anxiety, which affects my learning and concentrating. I am often labeled as ADD and ADHD by my teachers and put in small classes. My guidance counselor keeps suggesting that they put me in BOCES or a trade school. My mom always insisted that she was never going to do that and I will go to college.

She took me to all kinds of doctors for my chronic ADD condition and headaches. Thank God for soccer because I loved running up and down the field and was always determined to score goals even if it even meant running the opposite way once in a while.

When I was seven my ADD condition started affecting my ability to learn and this neurologist put me on medication for my disorder and my attention improved but I got more headaches and had a severe reaction to the meds, which made me itch and scream like crazy. The pediatrician said to stop the medication, and then for about six years I kept seeing doctors but nobody had any good answers. I kept up soccer and Girl Scouts and tried hard in school.

When we moved to Pennsylvania it was hard to make new friends and I still had headaches so this doctor had me do an MRI but the results were negative. I had to do this special diet and it kind of helped but not really that much. We moved back to Long Island because my dad was commuting so long every day and that was not good for any of us. My parents thought it would be more calm for me to live in the country in Pennsylvania, but I don't know if that made a difference, but anyway we came back to New York and then I got really bad anxiety.

I don't understand why my counselor has such little confidence in me. Many of my teachers tell my mom that they think I have ADHD or that I should be tested. All I know is I have trouble concentrating in class and I have a lot of anxiety. I get so mad at myself. How come I can't concentrate and why do I have trouble learning? I love to learn, but for some reason it doesn't reflect in my grades.

I hate myself.

June 2009

Freshmen year came to an end quicker than I thought. It was very tough for me because I was always feeling uncomfortable. Sometimes it would get really bad and finally my parents had to bring me to a doctor. I found out later that I had a chemical imbalance. This caused symptoms like a racing heart, and feeling uncomfortable and very warm. This was all part of anxiety.

Even now I still dislike that word so much.

Anxiety.

I don't want to think about that word.

Later on, I had to keep taking medicine to help reduce the problem. But it's not as easy as it sounds, like you just don't take a pill and your problems go away. Sometimes I would be switching medication every couple of weeks because some pills would increase my anxiety and that was very hard on me.

During the summer my family struggled to find a

house. It was always the same problem. People decided they wanted to keep their house and backed out of the deal or this other house was too small or too big or something wasn't right. I mostly played soccer in the summer with a travel team and focused on treating my anxiety. It felt good to be back on the field because I could relieve my stress and I didn't have to worry about anything else.

But we were getting desperate to find a house. Time was running out and my school had a rule that if you didn't live in the district you would be charged tuition for your child. The tuition fine would be $30,000! How could they really do that? Do they think people actually have money for that?

Summer was almost over and we were almost out of time. Our last option was renting a floor in an apartment house. This meant that the rest of our belongings had to be stored in a truck somewhere. I was relieved that my parents didn't have to worry about a bill from the school but I felt upset for my grandma because she was losing her company. To be honest, though, we had to get out of there because there was growing tension. I felt partially responsible because of my anxiety problem. During the night I would get anxiety attacks or symptoms of one.

It feels like I'm a basket case and my parents have to keep all of their attention on me to figure out what is happening because I've never been able to deal with anxiety attacks. I feel like I am steering or delaying the process of my parents trying to get everything straightened out, like our housing situation and just relaxing after coming home from their jobs. But not with me, with my anxiety. There is always something occurring with me that I feel like all of the attention is on me and it just feels unfair in my head, or at least that's the way I am thinking about it. And thinking about it like this just makes it worse.

I get so overwhelmed that it creates tension between my parents and sometimes my dad leaves my grandma's apartment to get some air. Anyway, we arrived at a rundown house where we would have to stay. I guess it was better because it was either get fined or live in this apartment. My sister and I shared a small room.

Once we moved in some of the tension decreased but not all of it. School was starting soon and it would be back to the same routine. My sister Alisa would be attending her second year of college at Dowling. I always thought she was so brave because she never really complained and I never witnessed her backing away from a challenge. Sometimes I wish I were like her because she is a strong-hearted person and obviously she doesn't have anxiety.

My sister always treats me well. Even though there is a four-year age gap we still did things together and always make each other laugh. I looked up to her as a kid and would always follow what she did.

Sometimes we were the typical family with a mini-van and all that. I think we went through three or four and me and my sister hated them. We would never sit still in our seats when my mom would be driving us to places when we were really little. We would throw our food at our mom from the way-back seat. We threw hamburgers, nuggets, and shoes at her when she was driving. We thought it was the funniest thing.

One birthday, my sister had me and her friends dress up as the Spice Girls and had a party. My sister is great. She always tried to invite me into her own plans.

September 2009

It was the first day of school and this time I didn't have to wake up at 4:30 in the morning. I would be taking the bus for the first time ever and my anxiety started to kick in again.

I hate feeling so uncomfortable in my own skin.

I think like this a lot.

The good news is, I was excited to go back to school because I had a little more awareness about what was going on there. I developed a system in my head about each class. The freshmen were scared of everybody. The sophomores thought they were better then everybody. The juniors thought they were tough. And the seniors were carefree because they just couldn't wait to get out of there and graduate.

This year I am a sophomore!

I tried out for the soccer team again at school and playing with the girls really helped to relieve my anxiety.

I made some friends here and there but I never invited them over to our house. I didn't want them to see where I lived or have to explain another story.

It would probably go something like this:

Oh, why are you living here?

Why can't you find a house?

Where are you from again?

Whatever.

October 2009

Soccer season is almost over. This month is getting tougher and tougher because I have to keep switching my medication. From here on, things could only get worse.

I was in biology class when my anxiety hit me like a ton of bricks, going through me stronger than ever. I had to stay after class and I told my teacher Ms. Coffey I thought I was going to hurt myself. In the afternoon I had to be taken out of class, then out of school, and then my mom had only one option, which was to bring me to the hospital. I had never been to a hospital for anxiety and I didn't even know you could go to the hospital for something like that. What would they do for me? Give me medication and then I could go home?

I've only ever been to the hospital on two occasions, when I was born and when I had a bad case of the chicken pox. My parents were standoffish about bringing me to the emergency room for something like this. My mom has some insight about these situations because she worked as a psychiatric nurse for many years. The only reason I went to the hospital is because I told the school I felt like I was going to jump in front of a car. School policy requires a student to seek immediate medical attention if they say something like that and since I didn't have a doctor for this sort of thing I had be taken to the hospital right away.

I couldn't go back to school even if I wanted to because the school wouldn't let me. That night I was rushed to the emergency room or the psychiatric center for children. I was interviewed by a social worker in a small room and she kept asking me the same questions.

Have you ever thought of committing suicide?

Have you ever harmed yourself?

Have you ever had dark thoughts about life?

No. Why is she asking me these questions.

It kept going on and on for the rest of the night.

I really wanted to punch this social work lady in the face because she wanted direct eye contact all the time and when I'd look away she'd say "right here" and put her finger on her nose. Why was she asking me if I wanted to hurt myself? Idiot—that would hurt and I don't want to cause harm to myself because I do not like being in pain!

When I was admitted to the hospital I was crying hysterically, and my family was, too. They couldn't do anything for me and I was basically alone, needing to be rescued. The doctors kept telling them all they could do is wait. According to the law, they would have to wait 72 hours and then they could write a letter trying to release me back home.

I was escorted behind two big solid doors, looking back, watching my family crying, and all I wanted to do was scream and kick. But I didn't because I knew that would only make things worse. Once I was on the other side of the doors the nurses made me take off my belt. I guess they thought it would be dangerous to me and the other kids. They took my clothes and made me wear this gown that looked like a tablecloth.

While you're at it, why don't you just take my hair out, too?

The inside looked pretty normal. It had a den area with games and movies. Down the hall were bedrooms, a kitchen, and small rooms with desks for us do class work.

Really? I'm in a freaking hospital and they are going to give me work to do?

Is this what they do on the cancer unit? They give homework?

What kind of messed up shit was this? I was going to have homework and assignments to do from school.

I was put in a room with another girl and I couldn't sleep the whole night. I was tossing and turning, crying my eyes out because I wanted to go home. I kept trying to focus on my family but that made me cry even more. I thought I was going to die right then and there. I couldn't understand how I could let this happen. I kept thinking it was my teacher's fault, but I knew blaming her wouldn't make things better. Ms. Boffey was just doing her job and obviously couldn't ignore a thing like this when a student tells her something like I did.

In the morning, we were called to breakfast. I didn't want to leave my room because I was so deprived of sleep and I missed my family. They told me I had to come because nobody could eat until everybody was present. I always had it in my mind that hospital food was gross but the breakfast was actually good. After we ate the nurse told us how the schedule was going to go. For the rest of the kids it was a normal routine and they already knew what to do. A doctor comes to check on us once a day and give us our individual medicine. The nurse said I could call my family and I would get two phone calls a day. I felt like screaming at her.

Wow, two calls, are you sure?

This comment was way too sarcastic and of course I didn't say it.

I felt like I was in a prison waiting for my parents to set me free.

I hurried to call my family and talked to my mom, dad, and then to my sister for about ten minutes. It was

27

hard to get what they were saying because some of the words were between sobs. I kept wishing I could jump through the phone and just be smothered by all of them. My mom told me she called my doctor who prescribed my medicine and he would call the hospital to help resolve everything. I talked to my sister about general stuff, like what they did today and what is prison like. I mean the hospital. When my time was up, I told them I loved them and they said they would try to get me out in another day.

I joined the other kids in a therapy session, which was new for me but for the other kids it seemed normal. We talked about why we were there, about our life, and what we would like to do when we made it out.

I keep talking like I was in an actual prison but that's because I didn't take it lightly being in there. I'm also a dramatic person and I've always been. Some of the kids' stories were really intense. I guess I didn't have it so bad. Then before I knew it, it was my turn to talk. I tried to be strong and I didn't want to talk for long because I knew it would lead to crying. I just quickly shared why I was there and ended with I want to go home to my family.

After the therapy session we went to the classroom and worked on our homework, which was sent from our schools. I found it interesting that they had an actual teacher working there. She was nice and helpful.

Do people in my school know where I am right now?

Did my teacher tell other teachers?

I kept getting worried thoughts and they kept going on while I was trying to do my work so I was having trouble concentrating.

If everybody knows, they might think I'm crazy.

I can't go back now. I can't go back to school.

Right in the middle of that biology class I had this, let's call it an "episode." I wasn't there with a bunch of geniuses, but the other students must have known something was wrong with me. I had my head down and my teacher Mrs. Coffey was next to me probably because she thought I was going to jump out the window. I don't know what she thought but she had to sit with me because the bell rang and the other students went about their day taking one last look at me before leaving for their next class. I had to stay right there until my parents arrived so I could be released into their custody.

How could I go back there?

The next day in the hospital it was the same routine: breakfast, therapy, school, and a visit from a dog! After the usual activities we got to relax and pet some dogs. It's more interesting then it sounds. It was actually really fun!

When we got back to our rooms the doctor came to check on us as usual and the nurse told me I had gotten a call from my family. After lunch I called them back but I didn't have any emotions in me to talk. But my mom had great news and I found out that tomorrow I would be out of the hospital!

The next couple of hours were rough. I couldn't sleep because I couldn't contain my excitement of getting out of this crazy place. I moved around in my bed and just thought of what I would probably be doing if I were home. I would probably be playing with my dog, watching TV, playing Sims 2 on my computer, or hanging out with my family.

The next morning, I felt light on my feet because by lunch I'd be gone. The rest of the day went by very slow. I tried not to look at the clock because if I did it would only make the day go by slower. I kept thinking about my teachers and the kids in my class. I hope they didn't think I died or something. I didn't realize I had been out for only two and a half days. To me, it felt much longer.

We got a little free time and went in the den. I kept to myself and didn't talk to anyone. I was excited to get out of this prison, see my family, and go back to school. We did one last therapy session and then it was off to lunch. I briefly talked about going home but I didn't want to make the other kids mad. Some were giving me jealous looks and I felt bad because one girl was going to move to a different building.

Lunch was good. We could choose between three different meals. I chose a hamburger with French fries.

Surprisingly, I didn't have to complain about the food because I'm a picky eater. After lunch, I counted down the minutes in my head and soon my parents showed up! I was trying not to cry or shake because I didn't want to look suspicious, but I was really excited to see them! The nurses said their quick goodbye's and gave me everything but my belt.

Well, whatever it takes to get out of here. Let them keep it.

I looked back at the other kids and sprinted out the door. The huge, solid door that had been guarding me inside was now behind me. I took a deep breath and ran to my family to be comforted. What I learned from this experience is that I would have to take more medication because on top of having anxiety I also had depression, which I guess is being sad but more intense.

The doctors told me that anxiety is part of depression or it had developed into it. People always say that with depression there is anxiety and vice versa.

To know I finally had a reason to be feeling this way was comforting and taking medication could help me feel less depressed. I felt better knowing that I wasn't some crazy kamikaze pilot flying off course and actually had some illness.

The psychiatrist put me on Concerta because he felt I was having anxiety because I couldn't focus in school. The neurologist ordered an MRI of my brain and the results were negative again. But soon the Concerta increased my anxiety and they took me off this medication just before the summer.

After we left the hospital I jumped into the car and put the seat belt on very tightly. I put my mom's bag on one side of me and whatever else was in the car went on my other side. It was like being tucked in between two walls so I couldn't get out. My parents didn't say anything. They just smiled and my mom held my hand. My dad said they were going to treat me to some lunch at Applebee's and although I already ate I didn't mind.

I didn't talk very much about the hospital. I didn't want to and I had no reason to, either.

When I got back to our apartment I ran inside and started hugging everything inside talking to myself.

Hello, crappy door!

Hello, small and smelly bedroom.

I was excited to be back, even in this temporary home. My sister was at class and I couldn't wait to see her because I haven't seen her either for two days! I ran to my dog Abbey and hugged her to death and even swore she started whimpering a little. My sister had made me a sign that said welcome home and I felt so relieved to be there, and she is such a good sister!

The next week I went back to school and things were pretty normal. Before I left, my mom told me that if I ever felt the way I did I should go straight to the nurse and say I was sick, then she would pick me up. I didn't want to take any chances, so when people asked me where I was I just said I was sick and that's that. In Ms. Coffey's biology class I didn't say much and I was scared, too. I didn't know how much she knew or if she told any other teachers. When the kids asked, I just told them the same thing—that I was sick.

June 2010

The summer after my sophomore year we found a house! Actually, as I keep telling my family, it was me who found us a house. One a summer afternoon, when we weren't even trying, we drove through Holbrook and I just spotted a house on this street we had never seen before. I thought it was odd because it was on a busy road and we were always looking at different houses in that town. We looked at it and liked it, and moved in during the middle of the summer.

The house was beautiful, mostly because it was finally ours, and I got the big room this time because it was my turn. It needed a little work inside but we were just excited to be in our own home. Can you believe the previous owner left us his entertainment center and his working lawn mower? He wasn't going to have any room in his new apartment so he left it to us.

My mom and dad wanted to have a family BBQ for

our two families to come see our new home. I helped my dad prepare by helping to fix up the backyard, and we called a service to come open the pool and they did a great job making it look like it was sparkling new.

The next day, my dad and I bought all of these cool floats and got a volley ball net for the backyard. The next week, we had our party and all of our family came. Everybody loved our new house and we all had a lot of fun. Then we lit off some fireworks in the backyard and watched from our deck. It was a great way to celebrate the 4th of July.

August 2010

I got an offer to be an assistant coach for a U-12 girls' soccer team! My old trainer Bart put in a good word for me with the coach. I started right away going two days a week. I was a little nervous. I guess anybody would be starting a new job, but of course I made it worse than it had to be. When I have to start something new I always over-think it and then I terrify myself.

I pushed myself to go with my mom's help and she dropped me off and left. The practice was a lot of fun, the girls seemed to look up to me, and I realized I was pretty good with kids. Three weeks into the season the girls became my buddies and when they see me they all come and jump on me. I feel like an older sister to them, and I've learned that I really enjoy working with kids.

The head coach, who has taught me a lot, offered me a job helping to train the team during the winter in an indoor soccer complex. I am real excited because this means I will have another job, but it also means I can't play school soccer again.

I had a long debate going on in my mind because I think too much and sometimes it gets annoying because I can't see what's going on in front of me. I decided to take the coaching job because that's what I know I want to do more. I figure senior year for sure I will play soccer.

The summer is coming to an end and almost all of our stuff is unpacked in our house. School is starting in a few days and I am excited, no longer nervous about it, but I still have an anxiety problem, even though I am doing a little better.

September 2010

I can't believe how fast the first two years of high school have gone and next year will be my last year! I still have mixed feelings about not playing school soccer because on one hand I know it will kill me inside to see the other girls wearing their jerseys in school. But on the other hand, I am happy because I know from people telling me junior year of high school is always the hardest and not playing school soccer may even make my junior year less stressful. I won't know until the middle of the year.

Today was the first day of school—again! My third year of high school and I can't believe it! One more year to go and then I will never have to come back to this place!

I arrived at school, pulled out my schedule, and headed to my first class. As usual, the first day was a waste of time because the teachers gave us a list of stuff we need for class. Then they gave us a survey thing like we're still in 7th grade and asked us our dislikes, activities, jobs, and what we liked to do.

First period I had media arts, which I found out later is the coolest class ever! We made cool projects, like movies, artwork, and pictures. The rest of my schedule was packed with regular classes. One class that would turn out to be my favorite was English.

That's mostly because I met a boy named Sergio.

He had a blue and yellow backpack that said Brazil on it. I love soccer, so when I saw that I made an effort to tell him, and then we started talking a lot in English class.

Oh, my gosh. I actually just met a boy I like and I think he likes me, too.

November 2010

I started to feel depressed out of nowhere. One day, I went to the school social worker and told her I felt like I was going to jump in front of a car. She immediately called my mom and told her what happened and then my parents took me to the emergency room. I was admitted to the children's psychiatrist center and the psychiatrist suggested that I take another type of antidepressant. My parents were totally against me taking medication because of all the bad effects they had on me. Anyway, I don't know how this happened, but they put me on Luvax and I guess that was okay.

How am I supposed to know what's okay?

December 2010

The semester and the year is almost over—thank goodness. I had my ups and downs with medication, school, and being in a psych ward, but at least Sergio is still my friend. I've known him for three months now and I think he still likes me so I guess that is a good sign because if I were him I would have thought I was crazy and stayed away.

I'm excited for the long holiday break but I'm also worried if I can handle it because something might happen to me if I don't stay occupied, especially when it gets too cold out or when there is a foot of snow and I will feel imprisoned in my own house.

That's one thing I hate about winter on Long Island. We get hit with a foot or more of snow unexpectedly and I get stuck in the house. I get depressed in the winter and wish I could go into hibernation until about February, but even then it's still cold and we get snow.

I will try to keep myself occupied by watching corny Christmas and romance movies on the Hallmark channel, which I am a sucker for all the time. Thank goodness for Kate McKinnon. She is my favorite person on *Saturday Night Live*. I can watch her videos and the show on YouTube and it always makes me feel less depressed.

I will keep coaching soccer indoors and this helps me keep active and I make some money, which is nice. I wish there was some retreat for depressed people to go to during the winter indoors—like a camp! A camp for people with mental illness for the winter there could be crafts, games, and team building—this is something I should create.

March 2011

I think I love Sergio.

I don't know who asked who, but our first date was bowling. I was so nervous I felt like things were moving around in my stomach. I guess that's what butterflies feel like. We had so much fun and we talked for hours. At the end, when I was waiting for my mom, Sergio kissed me!

Does this mean you're my boyfriend?

I asked him that because I have never been in a relationship or know how they work so I just assumed when he kissed me that meant he was my boyfriend.

He said "Suuuure," and smiled.

I hope that was the right thing to do, but it must have been because after my mom picked me up he texted me.

"I miss you already haha."

We are going to be together forever.

Wait.

Is it possible for somebody at my age to fall in love?

Have I ever been in love?

Do I know what it even is?

These are the questions I have been asking myself.

Sergio is different than anyone I've ever met. He is caring, sensitive, honest, and most important he understands me. He understands what I go through and he knows I have anxiety. He helps me through it and never asks for anything in return. I can cancel plans with him when I'm going through an anxiety phase and he understands.

I can't believe how lucky I am to have somebody like him in my life. Maybe God has forgiven me for my hardships and has blessed me with Sergio. I still don't understand, but I just have to get over it and embrace it because I know good things happen to good people.

But my headaches and anxiety are still there and my mom has to pick me up from school a bunch of times when it's too much. She brought me back to the psychologist and he suggested I go on Prozac. I wasn't sure at all but the doctor was very persistent to put me on this medication.

April 2011

I can't fight these feelings. I'm growing weaker every day with anxiety and bad thoughts. I'm considering hurting myself. I think of the consequences for my family and a few friends, which makes me feel worse.

I really don't know why I am like this.

This is in my thoughts too much. How can I have a positive mindset. Everyone sees me as so happy and nice. I guess I am a good actress. How come this can be true?

It's hard to eat dinner because I'm looking at my reflection in the knife. In my head I hear, "Just do it." Don't you want it to be fast and over with? Will it hurt?

I'm scared that soon I will hit my lowest point and then go too far. I'm trying to think how my family would feel . . . it would kill me.

I really hope I make it.

June 2011

Anger. I can't make out why I'm angry. I thought today was okay. I mean I made it through a school day without going to the nurse. Every other day or week I'm at the nurse because of headaches. But they can't do much. They ask me if I want a cup of ice? I'm thinking, what the fuck is a cup of ice going to do for me? Apparently, this is given to students and they eat it like it's a five-star meal for their migraine.

I keep my own bottles of Tylenol and stuff at their office but I always run out.

Anyway angry, yes, I'm angry.

I guess I'm confused why. I wasn't chosen to be a senior mentor for next year by my English teachers. But of course douche bag idiots, snobs, stuck up, troublemaker guys in my class *were* picked. I don't know how because they think they're hot shit.

But I don't consider that a key point to why I'm

angry. Maybe because I'm out of coaching now, maybe, I don't know. This anger makes me not able to talk to my mom or express how I feel. It took me five hours just to tell her I don't feel well.

Although I don't know why … I think too much.

I told my mom a couple of times I was bipolar or depressed, I'm not sure. Not that I would take my own life, but in my head the one thought I get a lot if I'm mad is I should just jump off (fill in the blank) and then that gets me by.

Sometimes I think I was a mistake or my mind doesn't want me to be happy.

July 27, 2011

Today I had to go to Centereach High School to take a practice course for my stupid state science test. I entered the school and everyone was looking at me, like I stuck out like a sore thumb.

Well, this isn't going to turn out well.

But everything turned out okay. After the test, I went with my mom to take my grandma to her doctor's appointment. I waited in the car and was feeling negative as usual. I thought to myself that maybe the reason why I don't know what I want to do with my life is because I am not going to make it past the age of 18. Maybe my life ends short and tragically.

October 2011

October 21st I made it to 17 years old. I couldn't believe I made it another year. I've been through some pretty rough shit. I wasn't as broken as other kids. There have been a few overdoses with kids at school of so I didn't have it the worst but I still have my pile of drama.

Sergio and I are still together. I am still trying to figure him out in class. He is kinda quiet but we talk a lot and I still secretly love him even though I haven't known him for very long.

I love the fall because I can eat pumpkin flavored anything and watch Halloween movies on the Disney channel that I am way to mature for. I snuggle up in my blanket on the couch with a warm blanket and my dog Abbey and watch movies all day long and keep to myself.

I am a loner, but at least I am happy by myself and not crying like some typical girl, like in that song "All By Myself." Not me.

December 2011

Still trying to figure it out ... I've been on so many meds, I don't know if I'm thinking straight, all these anti-depressants and anti-anxiety drugs, anti, anti, how about something positive?

Look at this list—crazy! And it's only some of it.

Ativan

Celexa

Cymbalta

Klonopin

Lexipro

Trazodone

Paxil

Prozac

Wellburtin

Xanax

Zoloft

I'm only 17! Somebody help!

March 2012

If there was ever a month to hate it would be March. I hate it so much because it feels like the coldest month and the longest.

But I got my first car! It is a 2006 Rav 4. I love it. I saved up quite a bit of money over the years from birthdays, Christmas, and coaching soccer so my parents didn't have to help me out that much with the money.

I am so happy I don't have to take the bus to school anymore—I feel so cool. I felt embarrassed that I was a senior taking the bus when most of them drove. I understand not everybody is rich and can afford a car but I want to feel the same as everyone else. Although the parking lot is technically full at school I was still able to get a parking pass through what I call my "political asylum." I work in the principal's offices and they all know me. I maintain such a good reputation the principal gave me a parking pass and I can park my car in the lot.

April 2012

I got involved with the environmental club last year because I care about the environment but also because we took a trip to Dowling College and that's where my sister attends school so I felt relieved that I might see her and run to her if I need to hide. That's what I was thinking when I signed up because I remember I was going on and on in my head, thinking too much and scaring myself out of stuff. But when were are about to go on the trip I was still very nervous because I wasn't sure how it was going to go and other schools were going to be as this event, too, and I didn't want to stick out in any weird way.

One of the principals in my school named Mr. Smith was very nice to me and understood what I had been going through. On the bus I was a little nervous but I just kept telling myself everything was going to be okay, thinking that by the time we got there I would eventually have to believe it. I recognized two girls from my class and we developed a plan to stay together.

We arrived at Dowling, the most beautiful place I have ever seen. It looked like a castle. The buildings were big, very pretty, and it looked peaceful. We all walked together in this huge glass room where we were given Dowling bags, pens, and a $250 scholarship! I didn't know what I would do with it because I wasn't even thinking that far ahead yet. Ha ha! What do juniors in high school know, I can say now, being such a smart senior.

But when we got our stuff our plan to stay together failed because all the students were split up. I was put in a group with students from different schools. We were supposed to focus on how to increase Long Island "youth activism" and had to come up with ideas to help get more young people active in their communities. We each went around the table, saying who we were and our school. As time went on we each came up with some pretty good ideas, which later we would have to put together and present. I don't know how but I actually spoke a lot in the group, helping to come up with ideas. After an hour and a half all of us broke for lunch. I met up with the girls from my school and we ate together.

Then a nice man named Mr. Louis A. Medina approached us and gave us his card and said he was a social worker. I was like, "Oh great, another social worker." He told us he was also the director at a Suffolk County youth bureau. I recognized him because he came to speak at our school last year. He talked about some of the problems with youth and his own story.

After lunch, we went back into our groups for one last time. We had to put all of our ideas and information together and pick two people to present what we came up with. I didn't volunteer because I had never talked in front of people before or really at all, ever.

I wished one day I could speak in front of people because it would show me how confident I can be.

Each group went up one at a time and presented their ideas. When it was our group's turn I stood in the back where I couldn't be seen. Our two presenters spoke about what we did and I could tell we did pretty well because we were getting lots of questions. Some of the kids in our group answered and I just kept thinking someday, someday I would have the courage to speak.

After that, I told my mom about Mr. Medina—about his story, what he does, and the rest of the important stuff. I said I wanted to call him and join the CONGRESS FOR JUSTICE he had at his office. JUSTICE stood for JOIN US TOGETHER IN CREATING EQUALITY.

My parents thought it was a good idea because it could help me speak out more. That weekend I called his office and set up a meeting after school to meet him with my mom. She helped me pick out a nice outfit and I drove us to his office in Hauppauge. When we arrived we pulled up to a huge building. I could swear it was as big as the Empire State Building. Not really, but it seemed like it at the time. My mom and I took the elevator up and I was already nervous but she kept reassuring me everything would be fine. When we arrived on his floor there were many desks with people working.

I met Mr. Medina's secretary, Kathy, who was the nicest lady and I talked to her for a little while before she brought my mom and I in and Mr. Medina's office. It was huge and looked over the whole parking lot. He had many pictures hanging in his office, mostly of kids that he knew or helped in the past.

"Why are you here?"

That was his immediate question.

"Because I want to help people," I said.

I told him I remembered him speaking at my school and I was listening to what he said and I wanted to overcome my fear of speaking. I talked to Lou, who said I could call him that, and then Kathy, too, and I decided to join the "Congress" and intern in the summer. Once a week I would come to the office and Kathy would run the meetings. One of the events the students and I were working on was "Unity Day." This event would help engage students understand and promote diversity.

We worked on this event through the rest of the school year when I was a junior and during the summer. Each week we would meet and we started to put a theme together and ended up creating what we called "Walk Through the World."

Each student was given a continent to look up, research the information, and put it together. I created another activity called "Hands of Hope," where the students could create a hand and write down what they learned at the end of the event. Over the summer, I met this boy named Tireak who was also interning. We went with Mr. Medina to Suffolk Community College in Brentwood to look at the space in the gym. Lou introduced us to a lot of important people that summer. I was even becoming more comfortable with speaking.

The day of the event, which was in the fall of senior year, a lot of students came from different schools. Even my school came, but I didn't expect them to notice me. The other students and I were running the show, talking about the different continents and running our section. That day, we also met Steve Levy, the county executive. He spoke first and then we got to speak to him. I talked to him for a while about how he got into politics and about his job.

I was actually having an important conversation with a public figure.

Weeks went by after the event and we were still getting great feedback from students and the schools. Being involved with the Suffolk County Youth Bureau helped me get involved with another event called "Stand Up For the Homeless." At this event, I helped less fortunate families receive clothing, food, and other items they needed.

I learned a lot from the family I was paired up with because in reality they were just like anybody else. They didn't start out poor or ask for it. They were once a middle class family and the father got injured and couldn't work. From there it just progressed and the family couldn't provide for themselves. It was upsetting, but it made me more motivated to help them get what they needed.

During my time with the youth bureau I received two awards from Mr. Medina and from his church. I received the Youth Achievement Award from Suffolk County, and my two principals and two guidance counselors came to support me. That day, I spoke in front of 200 people, which I never thought I would be able to do. But that is because I had so much support from wonderful people, like my family. Whenever I would go to Mr. Medina's office to intern or go on outings with him, he would push me to talk to important people and bragged about how great I was. Once I'd start talking, I couldn't stop. I was really gaining my confidence!

Then I received a $500 scholarship from Mr. Medina's church for college.

All of these positive experiences have helped me to better myself in my education and in life. I've been able to branch out in school and get involved with numerous community service activities. After the four years I was involved with the youth bureau, Mr. Medina was laid off and I couldn't believe it. Although he was brought to a different position, I still didn't believe it. I even started a petition in school to try and get his job back. I sent out emails to my teachers and peers, but then I gave up. I just stopped. I am not sure why, but I never continued. But one thing I do know is that Lou has helped me out more than I could ever imagine. To have made it this far now, being a senior at Sachem North High School, I have more confidence.

May 2012

I only have a month left of school! After that I will have a long summer ahead of me. I want to make sure I have to keep myself busy so I won't think a lot. I will probably see Sergio a lot like I've always had. I will still be working at the bakery on weekends. During the summer, I will work my magic and send out some resumes.

I can't believe I am graduating next month!!!

June 2012

I graduated high school! That's an okay accomplishment. I say okay because the real accomplishment was surviving four years of extreme obstacles, like anxiety, depression, thoughts of suicide, and a creepy doctor.

The one good thing I got out of high school was meeting Sergio—

We're basically high school sweethearts.

I'm just so happy to be done. Looking back, I wish I could have had more friends and been invited to a typical party with under-age drinking and doing dumb things— just to get the full experience of high school and my teen years.

But I was not your average teenager..

August 2012

It's been two months since I graduated high school and I am about to become a freshman at Dowling College. I can't really put all that together in my mind, that I about to start college. I am excited but I am also terrified, which is triggering off my anxiety. My parents and I have agreed that I should visit my doctor before my first day, just to let him know how I am feeling.

I went last week. I sat in his office and I let him know how I was feeling. He asked me where my mom was because she usually comes with me. I replied that she's working so I came on my own.

I'm still uncertain how my doctor started this awkward conversation. All of a sudden he was asking me to dinner, explaining to me that I didn't know him very well and then he told me I didn't know anything about relationships.

What was going on here!

How could I not be thinking that?

I'm no doctor, but I'm pretty certain he wasn't supposed to be talking to me like this. I'm his patient. I wanted to escape as quickly as possible. He tried asking me out to dinner and for my number.

"How about I call you?" he said.

"I have to ask my parents," I said.

He gave me some quick answer, like why would you need to do that? My legs were shaking. I felt like I was going to pass out. All I wanted was my prescription and to get the heck out of his office.

"No, I will call you," I said.

He gave me my script. I looked at his secretary on the way out of his office and quickly said I will call to make another appointment.

Did that really just happen?

I felt so violated. I quickly thought of my sister because she was the closest to me. I drove right to her job and let her know I had to talk to her, that it was a emergency. I told her what happened and she was in complete shock. She gave me a drink of water and together we called my parents at home. My mom was furious, not at me, but at the doctor—as was my dad.

Long story short, I didn't go back. I never went back to that doctor. My parents claimed to have reported him to our insurance company, but nothing ever happened.

For a while, I blamed my parents in my head, even though I know it wasn't their fault, but I felt so violated that I thought he should have been investigated. I wanted him to be reported, because that way he could never do this to anyone else ever again.

He represents such an ugly part of my life.

Through my early teenage years he was the one who had me switching from one medicine to another, which only made me worse. He wasn't even a good doctor, and he never made me feel good, so why wasn't anything done to him?

September 2012

I started school at Dowling College and enjoyed going to college because I felt I was learning much more there than in high school. This is probably because I am able to choose the classes I want to take and I'm not forced to take classes I don't need, like algebra or earth science. Although things in school are going well, I am still battling anxiety and I have no doctor.

My parents are working hard, as usual, and searching for a new doctor and luckily they were able to find one.

Thank goodness she is a woman.

It's also beneficial that her office isn't too far from our home. After my first appointment, my parents and I agree that Dr. Iyer is a good doctor. She evaluated me and the goods news is I am going to make it. It's not like she could tell me I won't make it, like I'm going to die or something; but still, she is positive in what she says and how she says it.

Sometimes, medication hopping interferes with my studies but I don't let that stop me. I have such a wonderful support system at Dowling through their student services. I love Dowling because it is small and all of my classes are in one building and I receive a lot of extra help.

November 2012

I am starting to get worse. I am still in school, but I have started to become mentally unstable. My focus, concentration, mood, and appetite have begun to decrease. Weeks and weeks have gone by and I have continued to see Dr. Iyer once a week, and the only thing that bothers my family and I is that even though I am switching from medication to medication nothing has been working.

I am a mess.

I can't stop thinking this is true.

I am lost in my own body.

That's for sure.

I feel like I am losing the strength to go on.

December 2012

My depression took over.

I thought I was a victim of identity theft.

It was the first week of December and I had to withdraw from Dowling—temporarily— because I was nowhere up to functioning properly.

I didn't even get to finish my first semester of college.

I was a disappointment.

I'm a loser, I thought.

Look at everything I thought I had overcome, only to end up failing a few months later. I wasn't suicidal, but I was depressed, and that meant more appointments with Dr. Iyer, which was fine, I guess, because she has a really soothing voice and she smells nice.

January 2013

I hit rock bottom during this time and was at my worst. One afternoon, I decided to go to a yoga class down the street. I thought if I had pushed myself it would make me feel better, but that wasn't what happened. I was halfway into the class and had a breakdown.

A strange force took over my body.

My mouth wanted to scream but the words didn't come out. I wanted to run into a wall because my body felt completely numb. I thought I was possessed.

I excused myself from the class and talked to my yoga instructor in the lobby. I told her I wasn't feeling right and had to go. She could tell, she said. She could sense negative energy from me. I didn't know how or what she meant, but I was thinking, "Okay, sense whatever you want, but I'm getting the heck out of here."

After that, I raced home and from there I was on my way to the hospital.

I was having the most awful thoughts about suicide. It was all I could think about.

I have never felt as strongly about it as I was feeling then, and I didn't enjoy it. My parents took me right to the hospital and I had to see a different psychologist. I didn't get admitted that night because when I was asked questions I lied to the psychologist, telling him I didn't have suicidal thoughts.

I will never forget my first encounter being admitted into the hospital. I will always remember it—every detail of the experience. I'm not saying I have been scarred for life because I don't know that yet and maybe I won't be, but I will never forget an experience like that.

The only reason I didn't get admitted that night was because I lied to the psychologist and he believed me. Instead, I was referred to an outpatient clinic the next week. But I remained in my old ways of thinking. For example, I would say to myself, "If I watch this TV thing or do this activity it will get me to four p.m. when it was only like two p.m. I still got so caught up in my mind that I had no time to relax for myself. All I could do was worry if I wasn't doing something right in the moment and what would happen.

I hope I like this outpatient clinic.

I kept saying that because if I did I would be gone from eight a.m. to five p.m. My thinking process started with "the bus comes at eight in the morning and I will get home by six."

The next week, my dad and I had an appointment to check out the outpatient clinic and fill out paper work to get me started in the program. The building was new. Inside it was very clean, but I was a little nervous. My father and I filled out some papers and I met some social workers. This social worker thing was becoming a routine. I was assigned to my own counselor, a man named Sal, and he seemed nice. I expressed to him that I was a little nervous to be there, although I wasn't going to start until the next week. He understood why I was nervous, and he explained to me that it was okay and that I was in a safe place and there were people there to help me.

"You're going to meet people from all walks of life," he said.

That was the last thing he told me, but I wasn't sure at that point if it was a good thing or a bad thing. He told me to give it a shot, see how it goes, and if I didn't like it I didn't have to come back. The program was voluntary, so people would be in and out. It might be the same people on some days and different people on other days. I wasn't sure if I would like that

The next Monday was my first day of the program, and I was regretting going already. I just wanted to hide in my bed. But if I wanted to get better I had to start somewhere, so I guess this program was better than being in the hospital.

That morning I woke up happy. I had already had gotten ahead of myself.

Yes! This will keep me busy until five and then I can come home, relax and go to sleep.

I was supposed to be retraining my brain not to think so far ahead but it was going to take some time. It wasn't like a light switch and everything would be different. It would take some time for my way of thinking to change. I guess it's a lot of work to fix your brain.

I waited patiently for the bus to come and as soon as it pulled into my driveway I thought I wouldn't be able to go. I heard the horn alerting me that it was time and I was immediately struck with fear. The thoughts stated pouring in.

I wish I could die.

I wish I could die right now.

I hope this happens to me so I don't have to go.

I am thinking stuff like that, on and on. I struggled to tell myself I was strong enough to go and my father was the only one home at the time and was trying to help me until he convinced me I was going and had no choice.

When the bus driver came to the door I knew it was too late to run. He was a simple looking man, not very tall, about five feet or so, with blonde hair, and he was very nice. He explained to my father about the pickup and drop-off time and gave his number in case he had any questions.

I got on the bus, looked at my dad, and gave him the desperate look.

Thanks a lot.

That's what I was saying to him with my face.

I sat right behind the bus driver in the first seat on the left side of the bus. I quickly reached for my iPod and told myself I wasn't going to talk to anybody else and just keep my head down. The bus ride was long and the driver had to pick up other people.

When we arrived at the place, the other people ran off the bus, excited, like they were arriving at camp or something.

Maybe I'll really like this.

That's what I thought, that this could be a free ride for me, meaning it could be something to keep me busy for the day. I would get breakfast, lunch, transportation, and then I would just come home and relax.

But when I got off the bus I felt lost. I was scared to move. I was far from home and I didn't know what to do. The other people were nice. They told me to follow them, and they helped me adapt to the daily schedule. It wasn't until I actually walked onto the floor that I didn't want to cooperate with anybody and just wanted to hide.

There were people of all different ages and problems. Nothing I was dealing with was as serious as some of the other people. I knew this wasn't going to work out, because I was being put somewhere again where I didn't belong or needed to be.

This day is going to go so slow.

I was already saying that in my mind.

Throughout the day, I kept to myself. I played on my iPod, and took the activities they had as a joke. Some of them were worksheets about dealing with depression, anxiety, and coping skills. One was about different pills, for example, the drug Paxil is a kind of pill.

Oh yeah, like I need to know that.

That's what I thought and said to myself.

Those worksheets seemed pointless and I just wanted to go home. I was disappointed because I thought this place would help keep me busy for the next couple of weeks, but that's not what I was thinking.

I'm not coming back. I'm not coming back.

I kept thinking that I was back at square one.

The only good thing I got out of the program was being assigned a social worker, the man I met on the first day I came there with my dad. His name was Salvatore, but he said I could call him Sal. He seemed nice, like he was a very caring person. During the day, I spent time talking to him and I felt he was very easy to talk to. I told him I didn't feel comfortable being in the program and he agreed that I wasn't having the same serious issues as some of the other people. I remember him telling me the day I came in to register for the program that I was going to meet people from all walks of life in the program. When he first told me that I kind of just blew it off and thought nothing of it, but when I finally started I understood. There were people there for all different kinds of issues and I felt like the lucky one for once.

But I also felt like I was going to be stuck in the building for the rest of my life. The day was going by so slow and I felt I couldn't escape. I kept counting down until it was time to leave, and eventually I had only one activity left until lunch. I was done the worksheets for the day and now it was time for group therapy. Everybody introduced themselves and explained why they were there, and I was in shock hearing some of the stories.

Some issues I could relate to, but others were worse than mine. I wanted to cry for these people, and some of them made me feel scared and worried about if they could make it through their problems. I tried not to associate myself with their situations. I guess I was lucky I didn't have it as bad as them. I thought I was dealing with the worst. I don't know if this is a cliché or if I know exactly what the definition means, but anyway I think it's a cliché but it goes like this:

Somebody always has it worse than you.

I guess it's a cliché because it's so true.

When it was my turn I just introduced myself but I didn't share why I was there. They didn't need to know, and if I was going to come back the next day I wasn't going to tell them. But I had to play this game. I felt like if I would have said, "Yeah, I'm not coming back" then the doctor or one of the social workers would have said, "Oh well, you have to give it another day."

I didn't care, because I didn't belong there, and I intended on begging my parents not to make me go back.

After the group therapy, I ate something disgusting, known as hospital food. After that, it was time to leave.

Finally I will get out of this asylum.

As soon as I got through the door, I signed out, and raced to the elevator. I made it to the first floor, rushed to the bus, and took my seat right behind the bus driver. The ride felt like it would never end because I couldn't wait to get home. That night, I expressed to my parents that I didn't want to go back, that it wasn't the right place for me. I brought up meeting my social worker, Sal, and my parents said I should call him, that he was somebody I can talk to.

Long story short, I didn't go back.

My parents agreed I was old enough to decide. We agreed that I still needed some kind of outside therapy.

After a couple of long weeks, I started seeing Sal. I wasn't uncomfortable talking to him by myself, unlike my last doctor who was asking me out to dinner. Sometimes, I had good days with what I call "things to do," which didn't make me worried or anxious. Then other days were bad, when I didn't have anything to do, and where I was planning out every hour of the day, and then I was driving myself crazy. This was making me depressed, anxious, worried, and that's what I had to work on.

Some days, I felt I wasn't going to make it to the end of day.

I wish I could go into coma until things pick back up.

That's what I kept saying to myself, hoping things would change, like school, or work. Being in this program was ideal for winter break. I didn't like the feeling of having nothing to do. I kept wishing I could sleep weeks until it was time for me to do something. On top of that, I felt like I didn't have any energy to hang out with Sergio. He understood what I was dealing with, and he wished he could help me, and he tried to understand how to help me. It's not that I didn't want to see him, but I felt I was starting to become tired of people and I was becoming alienated from people and society itself.

Winter break and the winter in general is my weakness. The cold and having nothing to do always gets to me. I just want to be alone and wallow in my depression. I don't have the energy to entertain Sergio because of my mood. The only thing that we do is watch TV because it's too cold to go outside or else there is nothing to do because we don't have any money.

During this whole month I was in such desperation to find answers that one Sunday after church I went to confession—twice. First of all, I didn't even have any privacy! The sessions were held in the mass hall and I was sitting back to back to the priest. I wanted to be in one of those dark booths with a curtain! I didn't want to be seen, not that I was embarrassed, but I was about to tell my whole life story to a man as holy as it gets and I planned on starting out with a script in my head.

It would have gone something like this.

Oh father, I have sinned for more years than I have been alive. I am seeking answers and forgiveness for I believe I still deserve a seat in Heaven.

I could have started in 2008, when all my problems began.

If I had a private booth and a privacy screen this is how it would have gone. Instead, I was quiet and muttering my words like I was doing a bad audition for a commercial. I went twice to two different priests and told each of them what I call my West Side Story, from the start to the finish and everything in between, which I don't know if people would confess to God, such as me dealing with depression and attempting suicide.

I basically was given two short homilies. The most of what I got from them was that I needed to put my trust in God and attend church more. This didn't really help. If I followed through with their advice, would God magically heal me and would I never experience anxiety or depression again? I didn't buy it. I still prayed every night and went to church when I could, but the stuff I was dealing with was out of God's hands.

Some days when I am feeling really good and have an appointment with Dr. V., I don't have much to talk about. I write down a list of stuff to talk about because I don't want to go into an awkward silence. On my good days, I ask to cut my session short because I am feeling so well.

With my new medication, I am feeling really well! Maybe I don't need my therapy sessions because I'm not worried about every hour of every day. I feel like I am slowly getting my energy back. It's the end of January but I can't wait to return to school.

March 1, 2013

I was wrong about getting back to school because everything has taken a 90-degree spin. I am experiencing the worst paranoia ever and I never even had paranoia before. I have anxiety but nothing ever like this. It's like I am one of those people on TV you see building a bunker because they think the world is going to end. I can't be by myself. I am always hiding under my bed covers, my parents' covers, or hiding in my sweatshirt.

It's not even like I'm anxious or anything. I just feel overcome by fear and in my head the only way I know I am safe is under a comforter, not that this will protect me from a meteor or anything, but it's not called a comforter for nothing, right?

My parents thought I was sleeping walking one night but it turned out to be a seizure.

I think maybe this happened a bunch of times. I can't recall when I had them because I never had signs of an oncoming seizure, and I don't I have any memory of them after they happen. Before this, I never experienced a seizure, or I definitely did not have any knowledge about them. I thought of a seizure as like when people have a drug overdose.

I don't know how or why but suddenly they are occurring more. Some days I can't stop shaking and my parents don't know why. This started another journey of visits to the hospital and one day I was brought to the emergency room because I was shaking uncontrollably when another seizure happened and one of the doctors actually got to witness it.

I was in the emergency room. Doctors did simple tests on me, like closing my eyes and touching my nose, lifting my legs, and other stuff. It was strange. I think I failed most of the tests because I couldn't touch my nose, I couldn't walk very well, and the left side of my leg was very weak. This meant more doctors' appointments, and nobody could pick up what was going on with me. It got worse with my anxiety coming back so my mom brought me to a neurologist.

After seeing a neurologist I was put on another medication for seizures.

"Don't be surprised if your anxiety and paranoia goes away while you're on this medicine," the doctor said.

Hold on there, pal, you must be joking.

I was thinking that to myself, that no anxiety and feeling normal for once was too good to be true. But it turns out he was right.

I feel like a new person. I started working on the weekends again at the bakery, and I feel amazing! I feel so good I started looking for another job, a little something extra, maybe some volunteer work, just to keep me busy during the week.

I don't remember exactly how it came about, but two weeks after I started this new medicine I began to volunteer at an assisted living center down the street from my house. The assisted living home isn't just a nursing home. It's a community for older people with dementia and Alzheimer's. I put myself up to the challenge and I met with the activities director. I didn't really understand the concept of dementia and Alzheimer's. The director explained it to me and truthfully I was nervous because I wasn't sure I knew what I was getting myself into.

One thing I knew is I love helping others and I am great at it. I am calling bingo some days, playing board games, and I even brought in some of my crafts as prizes for people playing the games.

March 10, 2013

After this happened, my dad knew something was really wrong. I was home one day—well, I was home many days during this time, because I wasn't going to school.

Anyway!

I was bored and decided to take my dog, Abbey, for a walk. She's in dog heaven now, but she was my first dog as a kid and I loved her.

Where am I going with this?

Okay, so I decided to take her for a walk and I made it down the block to the stop sign. Long story short, I didn't come back with Abbey. I walked right into the house without her.

"Nicole!" my dad said. "Where's the dog?!?"

What is he talking about? Abbey is in the house! Why is he so worried?

I was convinced that my dog was in the house and had no memory of anything else.

You probably understand where this is going. I must've had a seizure and dropped the leash and walked back home without a clue that I left Abbey at the stop sign on a busy road. I ran back down the block, confused out of my mind after sitting on the couch. Luckily, my dog was sitting at the stop sign, looking at the clouds as if she were waiting for a bus!

I'm very lucky nobody kidnapped her. I'm lucky I didn't get hit by a car, too!

I thought it was the funniest thing because I really tried to defend my innocence to my dad, saying Abbey was in the house when I had actually had a seizure and ditched her outside.

That's what I was thinking because the truth was way too weird.

Mid-March 2013

The staff really appreciates my help as well as the residents, and although I'm not getting paid I don't mind it! I think helping others in need is something better than getting paid for it, and maybe in the future I can get paid.

I am still doing really well after getting the medicine for seizures but my parents and I still question why all of a sudden a healthy girl was getting seizures in the first place. This is something that has to be looked into more because I am already on enough medication as is.

This started a whole round of visiting doctors, starting from my general doctor, to get blood work, a spinal tap, which is the most uncomfortable thing I've ever had. They didn't even put me asleep, which I think is just rude!

My mom took me to Mather Hospital to get blood work and we were sitting in the office and the first thing the nurse said when she walked in was "Bagel store!"

I just shook my head.

Really? I work in a local bakery and now I get recognized as "bagel store?"

Hello? I have a name.

She was like, "Oh you work at the bagel store," and yakity yak yak.

Okay lady, forget about your freaking bagels and take my blood!

My parents and I visited my neurologist and he recommended another MRI so my mother and I took another visit to Suffolk County Radiology to get my test done. The same day, my doctor called me to come in because he wanted to see the results immediately. I sat in his office for the longest time. He gave me small tests, like walking, touching my nose with my eyes closed, and tested my strength. I still failed. I could not walk right, or touch my nose, or show any strength in the left side of my leg.

The doctor put the CD of the results in the computer and scanned both pictures of my brain. I wasn't trained to read them, but as I looked from my seat I saw something I've never seen before. I saw two dark pictures of my brain, but I guess somebody who isn't trained can't read them. I sure knew I couldn't. The doctor also put the scans up to the light, comparing the pictures of my brain.

This was the longest appointment ever!

He was looking at the images and I just wanted to scream, "AM I GONNA DIE?"

The way he examined them, with this questioning look on his face, and in his eyes, I knew something was wrong, like he had discovered the treasure on a map. The doctor had told us he thought he found something off, but just to make sure he called the people at Suffolk County Radiology who read the MRI and then he confirmed with them that there was a problem.

You better be right you stupid-idiot because this is my freakin brain you're talking about!

That's what I was thinking.

The neurologist finally hit us with the news, that there was a tumor on the right side of my brain and some sort of epileptic tissue. He told my mom and me that I was going to need surgery—no doubt about that.

My mom's face said it all, like she had just been hit by a truck.

She takes a deep breath and says "alright" to the doctor—just that one word—like when something is distinguished as a fact, and since it's a fact that's that. She didn't cry, she was calm and collected.

How could my mom be so calm?

My doctor just told me I have some ball sitting on the inside of my brain that is giving me seizures and her response is "alright?"

I limped out of his office into the waiting room, crying. I couldn't believe the change of events. I thought maybe I was sick with a virus but now I needed brain surgery. Before I left, the neurologist assured me everything was going to be okay.

Easy for him to say, he probably says that to everybody.

April 29, 2013

Long story short, I had to leave Dowling College in mid-semester. My neurologist referred me to one of the best surgeons in New York City.

"If you're going to get this done, I want you to have the best," he said.

Yeah, me, too.

On the train ride there with my parents, a guy turned his head to me and said, "Can I have a whole wheat bagel with cream cheese?"

He must've been a regular at the bakery and recognized me.

Stupid ass bagels!

I was really annoyed. I jokingly said to my parents that I was quitting after this.

May 2, 2013

Everything is happening so fast.

The next week after I saw the neurologist, I was at an epilepsy center in New York City. My parents questioned if I could handle being on the train because they obviously didn't want me having a seizure on the Long Island Railroad. After we arrived at Penn Station, we had to take a cab to the office. I wouldn't have minded walking but I would be limping so we agreed it was best to get a cab.

I couldn't remember the last time I was in New York City. All the buildings were tall enough to reach beyond the clouds, and the streets were busy with car horns beeping every second, one after another. The buildings looked fake from a distance, like if somebody was driving into the city they wouldn't look real, but up close they were as real as could be.

Whenever I would visit the city I would always be

annoyed when I first got there by the loud noise, smells, and crowds, but afterward you appreciate what the city has to offer. I enjoyed the scenery, the stores, and the walking. When we arrived to the office I only had to wait five minutes until the doctor came in—the shortest I ever had to wait for a doctor, but it was the longest five minutes of my life.

I was honestly so scared. I never had surgery before, and I wasn't sure what to expect.

The doctor came in and he introduced himself as Dr. Werner Doyle, who was going to be my surgeon. I never met a doctor like him. He was funny, compassionate, and really nice. He really cared, and he explained stuff that was going on. He didn't care about the time. He went into full detail of how my brain was working and what was causing these seizures. He agreed that surgery had to be done as soon as possible.

Unfortunately, my dad was going to be out of a job at the end of the month and would only have his health insurance for a certain amount of time. My parents explained to Dr. Doyle and his staff about the situation and they tried to straighten things out.

Dr. Doyle's nurses, Allison and Mary, made phone calls to NYU hospital to try and get me a hospital bed because the sooner I could get admitted the quicker I could be assessed and have surgery.

After an hour of working with insurance, phone calls, and waiting, we had to wait some more. The nurses were working on getting me a bed at the hospital, but it was going to take some time so instead of waiting at the office, we grabbed a bite to eat and did some shopping. I wasn't prepared to stay overnight at a hospital so I bought some things I needed. I thought I was just going for an appointment. I didn't realize I would be checking into a hotel for the next four weeks. My parents bought me what I needed: toothpaste, a hairbrush, clothing, definitely clothing like underwear! If I was going to be miserable I didn't want to be gross, too. I'm just kidding, so after killing four hours of waiting we finally got a call from Dr. Doyle's nurses and they said they had a bed ready for me.

After a chat with Dr. Doyle, his staff sent me right over to NYU Hospital. If there was any hospital that was the best of the best—in my opinion this was the one. The hospital wasn't very far at all from Dr. Doyle's office and it was unlike any hospital I've ever seen before, and if anybody has been to many hospitals it is me.

NYU hospital is amazing! If I were to just come in to use the bathroom, not even knowing it was a hospital, I would probably think it was a five-star hotel. The doctors couldn't quite get me to the epilepsy floor yet because there wasn't a bed available so I was in the emergency room for a couple of hours. I didn't mind being there because honestly I was used to it by now with all of the trips I have made to ERs.

This time it was a little different. I tried to relax by watching TV. I thought it would keep me busy for a couple of hours but I was wrong. It had 40 channels, but only ten worked, and the rest were in Spanish or they didn't come in. On top of that, I had an old lady screaming next to me! She was complaining because my TV was too loud, She kept saying, "Tell her to use her headphones, somebody give her headphones for her TV!" I think she was also jealous because the doctors and nurses were giving me more attention. She didn't have any severe problems, but I'm pretty sure she was hallucinating. The woman had an amputated leg, and she kept screaming for medicine, and saying that nobody was helping her and they were all trying to kill her.

An hour of this and she never stopped.

After another hour and a half all I was doing was crying because I didn't understand why she was acting so crazy and screaming. Two hours went by, maybe, I don't remember. My parents said I had a seizure. They said it was a strong one because after the seizure I passed out. The doctors in the emergency room agreed that they had to get this lady away from me because she was making me nervous and caused me to have a really strong seizure.

I finally made it to the epilepsy floor, it was much quieter, and there were people my age. Only a few were adults. I didn't talk much to the other patients because it wasn't a group setting.

The view from my room was beautiful, with the river to my left and buildings to my right. The room was very simple, with a bed, a TV, a closet, and a recliner seat. There was no privacy because I had a camera watching me. The only place I wouldn't be filmed was in the bathroom, but that's understandable because that is intrusive.

The day was very long. I kept having all different kinds of tests, and unfortunately my dad had to go on the train and get back to his job for the couple of days he had left. It was getting late in the night so my dad said his goodbyes, and he gave me a kiss on my head. My mom didn't want to leave me. The first couple of days she stayed with me, sleeping next to me on my bed and switching to the half-broken recliner in my room. I didn't get much sleep, although I don't know how anybody could in the situation I was in.

May 3, 2013

First thing in the morning, a nurse came into my room and told me I was going to be given an IV. I didn't mind. I had them in my arms before. When she brought out the IV though she wasn't going for my arm. She put it in my hand! If I ever experienced anything so painful in my life this was it. I had a small tube or needle sticking into the skin on the top of my hand. I have no idea why they put it in that spot.

As if I wasn't put in enough pain already, during my lunch another nurse came in to attach wires to my head!

After lunch, she came with her kit and started to work. The smell of the glue was strong, like when you go to the dentist and they give you the toothpaste that they claim is bubble gum flavor but tastes like rotten strawberries. It was that kind of smell but five times worse.

I say this with sarcasm. The good news is, these wires were going to be attached to my head for the weeks leading up to my surgery. On top of everything else, after she was done with her artwork of wires she wrapped a white cloth around my head, covering the wires. You might think it doesn't sound bad but it looked like a huge sweatband around my head. It was tight, and I looked like a nut job, and the worst part of it was I couldn't leave my room because the wires were attached to a box. The wires monitored my brain activity so the doctors could capture any seizure activity.

May 6, 2013

The first few days were torture because I was being watched. I couldn't get out of my room, and I was starting to lose my mind. As much as my mom wanted to stay with me, she couldn't keep sleeping on a broken recliner. I cried for the first few days and asked my mom why God was allowing this to happen to me.

What did I do to deserve this?

That's what I was asking.

My mom needed to rest. She told me she needed to be strong for me, and I couldn't quite understand what she meant. It was hard to find a hotel, and my mom didn't want to be too far from me, and a lot of the hotels were either too expensive or too far from the hospital. The different nurses told my mom to check with Dr. Doyle's team and with help from Allison and Mary they found my mom a room at a hotel not too far from the hospital, which was covered by the hospital foundation.

The next few days all I did was have tests of my cognitive abilities and walking down the halls with the box attached to my head. Eventually, the whole situation grew on me and like any difficult situation I used humor to get through it.

Whenever I needed to get up I was supposed to use this call bell on my wall and the nurses would see it on the camera and come down to help me. Instead, I'd just get up and disconnect the wires from the wall and plug them into the box so I could walk around my room or down the hall.

The nurses would jokingly say, "Where are you going Nicole?"

I'd say, "I'm going for a walk" and just grab my stuff and go.

I'd crack jokes with the nurses and sit by the window and watch people. I had some family visit me from Pennsylvania and I hated people seeing me like this but I didn't care—I just cracked more jokes.

I kept counting the days until my surgery because then I could finally take a shower, which by the way would be going on 1 week now since I showered. When the day comes for my surgery I would get these wires off that were glued to my head. Only a few more days and I could finally feel the freedom of moving around without being on a leash.

Even though my mom was in a hotel she wasn't too far because each morning I would wake up and she would be right next to me. I felt safe knowing she was next to me before I even woke up. I was starting to understand now what she meant by her being strong for me. She helped take care of me. She took me for tests during the day, and told me everything was going to be okay. I couldn't image a better mom. She had done so much for me, and she was making the time fly by faster being next to me.

May 9, 2013

I finally got the date of my surgery, and tomorrow I will be in the operation room. I don't think I will be able to sleep tonight.

I'm not sure what's come over me but I think reality has hit me. I am up all night, tossing and turning, thinking about how the next day will go.

I keep thinking the awful words "What if," which my mom has always told me never to think of. I keep wishing that something will go wrong in my surgery, for example, not waking up from anesthesia, or maybe my head bleeding.

Until this time I have never been scared. I guess it never really hit me—that they are going to cut my head open. I think I was just caught up of getting out of the hospital, and I guess I forgot the only way I would get out is if I had got the surgery done.

My surgeon Dr. Doyle came into my room and he

explained the possible effects of the surgery. It must be part of his job to explain the possible downsides of him ruining my life.

I'm joking.

I don't want to be in the room when he is talking about the procedure and percentages of things that could happen. That makes me feel so much better. Not!

May 10, 2013 — Before

I am so tired from struggling to face the reality that I am having brain surgery today. The good news is, my mom was right next to me as I woke up, I expressed to my mom how I was feeling and she assured me everything is going to be fine.

Really?

I didn't say anything, but I thought, how can she know that?

Are you a fortuneteller? How do you know everything is going to be okay?

It is obviously a parent's job to tell their child those famous words "everything is going to be okay." I don't know why I am thinking about it so much because I am going to be asleep, anyway, but I guess I have to think of the positives of having the surgery.

I can't eat breakfast, which is horrible because I am hungry. I've been starting to enjoy my hospital meals.

After I received my medicine, a doctor came in to detach me from the wires.

Freedom!

I couldn't stand the awful smell of the glue, and the wires were all tangled together around me like a spider web. After she finally finished, I was allowed to take a shower. I never went one whole week without taking a shower. I never felt so relieved to take a shower in my life, even if it was only going to be for a few minutes.

The hardest thing was trying to get the glue out of my hair. That's going to take a few more showers, but I got to get started. When I was done with my shower I walked back to my room and in my head I was saying to the other patients, "Sucker, I'm getting out of here!"

I watch some TV to pass the time because my surgery time is set for four in the afternoon. I am still not allowed to eat. The least they can give me is a piece of candy. At three I am past starvation, and I think I am going to pass out. My mom and I exchange looks and she takes my hand and says, "Nicole, everything is going to be fine, and you will be better after the surgery."

When it's almost four, two nurses come into my room with a stretcher. I joke around with them and say "take me away" with my arms open, like I am waiting for them to handcuff me. The nurses pull me on the stretcher through the hallways, which seem to go on forever.

It is almost time for me to go in. My mom gives me a kiss and promises me everything is going to be okay. She smiles at me and takes the elevator upstairs to wait for me. I am lying outside the operation room and then it hits me.

I am terrified.

I feel like I am in a twilight zone. I am in a basement, with doctors in lab coats, with masks on, and signs that say, "Caution. High something, blah, blah, blah." This is like lab talk to be careful because there is dangerous stuff going on.

I am overcome with fear like I never felt before.

I don't know what is going to happen.

Why am I doing this?

I go back in my mind to the night when Dr. Doyle explained the possible effects of having the surgery. I had to focus on the positives, like Dr. Doyle and my parents told me, that by having the surgery it could cure my anxiety and the depression I experience.

I went back to thinking about what my neurologist said to me in the doctor's office about the lesion in my brain causing the anxiety and depression. I can never fully understand everything, but it seems like I could have had this for a long time if it has been causing me anxiety for so much time.

"Are you ready?"

I am about to be taken into the operation room and a woman in a lab coat is asking me this question.

Yeah sure, just stick your fingers in my brain and have fun!

I felt like saying that. She has me wait a minute before she rolls me in on the stretcher and I close my eyes and say a prayer to God.

Please God, don't let me make it out of surgery. Can you have me not wake up or can I get internal bleeding and basically die?

I am scared because I don't know what is going to happen. I'd rather die in surgery than come out with something wrong with me, like I can't talk or something like a physical disability.

At this moment, I truly think God has the power to do this and I give him my consent to take my life.

May 10, 2013 — After

I woke up with the most horrible headache I've ever had. I had a bandage wrapped around my head and staples going down the right side of my head just above my ear. The doctors didn't use stitches. It was staples, like you see in a stapler but these were heavy duty.

I thought being surrounded by my family and even my Aunt Nancy by my side would be comforting but I couldn't enjoy it. I couldn't even open my eyes because of the pain I was in.

Why can't I have cancer instead? It's probably less painful.

I kept thinking that.

May 11, 2013

After a whole day in the emergency room I am back in my room, what I like to call my "jail cell." As soon I was put back here I am right in view of the cameras again and everybody is watching me. My mother and aunt stay with me during the day and try to comfort me. They brought me the best veggie burger I have ever had. Aunt Nancy and Mom are starting to enjoy the city. They enjoy the walking and have discovered a new restaurant they fell in love with and I want to go there, of course, but I can't.

Duh.

May 12, 2013

Different doctors keep coming into my room to introduce themselves as the ones who experimented on my brain. Today, I started some tests with one doctor to see how I was "functioning" I guess. I put blocks together, repeated words and numbers, and did some reading. It was very easy, annoying at times, but it kept me busy, and took most of the day.

I also had to practice walking, which makes me feel like a baby. For who knows what reason, when I was having the surgery something offset my balance. I start at one end of the hallway and a nurse at the other gestures to me to walk. I really hate this and I want to curse out the nurse. It isn't personal. It's just that I hate being treated like a baby.

I am 19 years old and I have difficulty walking!

I understand some people have a disability and they cannot walk, but I was a healthy person, at least physically, which made me think that walking should be second nature, or whatever that expression is, except that walking doesn't feel natural at all right now.

One of the social workers came and talked to me for a while to see how I am doing. The hospital has to do these tests to make sure I am stable and okay to eventually go home. As I talked with the social worker, he asked about how I arrived here, how it was affecting me, and my current state of mind.

I basically lied out of my ass.

I replied with "Yeah, sure" and answers like that, nodding, saying I was fine and I was positive and crap like that. I couldn't tell him the truth—not that I didn't want to, because I wanted to tell him, but I am sure that if I did or if I do now he will keep me here longer, or worse, he could send me to the psych floor.

The truth is, I am starting to lose it and I want to die.

I am stuck in my room, thinking about ways I could die quickly. I often look out the windows and consider jumping. I even walk by the windows once in a while to watch people on the street and just observe the city life. I am still being watched everywhere I go and sometimes when I am by the window I examine how thick the glass is, but unfortunately it is too thick. I keep thinking that if I try to jump through the glass I'll probably just bounce back from it because of how strong it is.

Some nights, I cry in my bed.

Why do I do to deserve this? Have I done something wrong in my life to be here?

That's what I am thinking a lot.

May 13, 2013

I have another MRI after my surgery. My surgeon and his staff come to visit me in my room and see how I am doing. Dr. Doyle sits with my parents and me and tells us the MRI came out good, and the tumor is removed. He tells me I am going to make a great recovery and everything is going to be much better for me.

Then Mary, a nurse on Dr. Doyle's team, crouches down next to me.

"I'm sorry, Nicole," she says, "but you never had ADD or ADHD. I'm sorry for what other doctors told you or diagnosed."

I had no words. I couldn't even process this.

The tumor could've developed at a young age, growing slowly and affecting everything inside me, so my doctors I had a learning disability, and teachers and staff doubted me at one point in high school, acting as if the only thing I would be able to do is flip pancakes.

My mom told me that as a kid she was always bringing me to different types of doctors to address my learning issues and difficulty concentrating. I was put on all the wrong medications, ones that made me manic, while this "thing" kept growing in my head, going unseen, so I never received the proper help. When really it was this thing growing in my head the whole time at a young age and it reached its full potential, finally causing me really bad issues.

My last day at the hospital feels like the longest ever. One of my nurses tells me to practice walking more to get my strength back, so my mom takes me around walking through the hallway. I still have some pain in my head, but it was expected because I just had major surgery.

My dad is on his way here from home because he decided we should drive in the car back to Long Island because the train might be too much for me. My mom is with Mary and Allison, signing release papers and going over a few things. I am holding onto the wall, practicing walking like a loon.

I must look like a lost person scaling the wall going up and down the hallway.

As I walk back and forth, some of the nurses are cheering me on.

"You're doing good Nicole!"

I want to say thanks and shut the hell up!

That's what I am thinking, but I just smile.

I just want to go home. I can't take it anymore. I never would have thought I would be in a situation like this. I am used to running! I played soccer my whole life, and as a kid my parents could never catch me. As soon as I got into a store I would find a way to get out of my stroller and I was off like lightning, and now, at 19 years old, I am practicing walking again.

As soon as my mom is done with the release forms my dad calls to let us know he is outside the hospital. My mom rolls me out to the car in a wheelchair, and as soon as I get outside I feel the air surrounding me. It's so good, like smelling a flower for the first time. It's a flower smell, like no other city air—not the greatest, but I am being released from the hospital!

The ride home is much longer then I imagined, probably because I keep telling myself it isn't real.

Nope, not there yet, don't get excited . . . still not there yet . . . don't get your hopes up!

When I finally arrive home it is pretty late, and the first thing I do is open the door and my dog immediately runs to me and jumps in my arms. She is whimpering and licking my face. Usually I might be a little grossed out, but I haven't seen her in four weeks so having my face covered in doggie breath is well worth it.

When I go into my room for the first time it doesn't

feel as if anything has changed. The first thing I do is lie in my bed, and as soon as I put my head on my pillow I fall right asleep.

After a short nap, I don't move. I'm not sure where I am.

I have to remind myself that I am no longer attached to wires. I have to survey my room to look for a camera that could be filming me, but I remember I never had one. I don't have to push a button to tell my mom or dad I am getting up to use the bathroom. I don't have to force hospital food down my mouth. I can enjoy my favorite homemade meal by my mom—lemon chicken. I feel like I am eating a meal at a restaurant, although I am completely familiar with the meal the taste seems to be different, better than anything I have ever tasted. I got so used to hospital food, I was like "holy shit" that chicken is great!

I call Sergio right away and he tries to act as if everything is okay since he last visited me at the hospital, but hearing his voice through the phone I can tell he is holding back sobs. I don't like making Sergio worry about me, but at the same time it is comforting. I never had somebody outside of my family care that much about me. I guess what I'm saying is, I never had a boyfriend that cared that much about me.

May 31, 2013

These past few weeks I have been in a lot of pain from headaches caused from my surgery. I'm glad it's over with, and the only thing I couldn't stand were the staples in the right side of my head, going down along to my ear. I have to take painkillers every day, which make me sleepy so I do cat naps. I am probably 20 pounds overweight with all of the medicines and napping, but there isn't much exercise I can do yet so I am staying out of bathing suits—for now. I don't want to be spending my whole summer like this, and I can't go back to work for a couple of weeks. I still have to go to a check up appointment in the city before I can even think about that stuff.

I am going to see Dr. Doyle soon and he will take these steel staples out of my head that is causing me all this pain. He asked my parents if I had a previous MRI test done before I ever had surgery. I thought it was an odd question, especially to be asking now.

My parents sighed, and then found a CD from Suffolk County Radiology from a year ago when I was experiencing migraines.

Something doesn't feel right.

June 10, 2013

I keep telling my parents on the way into the city to see Dr. Doyle that we are going to get in and get out and that's it, because according to me, there is no coming back home without me! My parents assure me I am going home with them, that I have nothing to worry about.

When we arrive at his office some of the staff recognize me and say hello.

Don't get used to it, I'm not staying!

That's what I am thinking in my mind.

Dr. Doyle removes the staples from my head and we show him the CD of my MRI from one year ago, as he requested. The doctor reads the results of the MRI and my parents and I can't believe what he is telling us. It turns out this MRI showed the tumor that Dr. Doyle had removed from my brain just weeks ago. I couldn't process that in my mind but I was sure I wasn't going to do anything about it because after a few weeks since the surgery my dad was still without a job and I was starting to doubt if I will ever get better. The pain in my head is still so severe that my parents have had to bring me to the emergency room a couple of times a month.

Although I still haven't experienced any anxiety since before my surgery, I can't stop my anxiety medicine. I don't know why. I mean I've been on 50 different medications and the one thing I don't have is anxiety, but I still have to take medicine for it.

June 15, 2013

I have an appointment with Dr. Iyer and I am sure I don't want to go. That's because of the obvious reason—I don't have anxiety!

I can't believe that a year ago all the anxiety and depression I ever had could have been fixed. I want to call the doctor out on this in her office.

How come you never looked into it?

I want to say that, but my mom told me to keep my mouth shut because she is going to look into it.

Dr. Iyer asks how I have been feeling, about the anxiety, and how I am handling everything. She is very nice, as usual, and smiling, but I feel so hopeless, like I am being used or something. I look at her and don't say anything out loud.

Damn well she knows I probably didn't have anything wrong with me.

In my mind I was thinking that.

I hadn't even finished my first semester of college because of the depression and anxiety, and I was put into an out-patient clinic for these problems and I never actually had any of them, not really.

Maybe I did. This is confusing. Maybe I didn't. I didn't.

If it weren't for the seizures I would have never known I had a tumor in my brain. My mom did what she could, looking into lawyers about my missed MRI and the fact that I was misdiagnosed, but there was nothing anybody could do.

At least that's what they say.

My dad continues going on interviews and also taking an online class to learn more of the complicated stuff he went to school for. I am struggling to accept that nothing can be done about my MRI or that I was misdiagnosed.

I am getting so caught up in it that one night everything finally hits me. I go into my room and I feel as if I am stuck in a bad dream. I crawl into my bed, I start to cry, and it goes on for an hour. I recall everything, like I am still in the hospital, like I never left. I don't think it was fair what I went through. Now, even the lawyers can't help me. I was away from home for weeks. I couldn't even walk, and I had freaking brain surgery, and I am still on medicine I don't even need for problems I haven't ever had. On top of that, I'm huge.

This is fucked.

I go downstairs to get water with my face all red and tears streaming from my eyes. My sister and mom are on the couch.

"Nick what's wrong?" my sister says.

I can't answer, and I go back upstairs. I am thinking, here is the "problem of the day" and it's who will be the one to follow me and comfort me? I wasn't surprised when five minutes later my mom walks in to my room and sits right next to me on my bed. She asks me what was wrong.

Here we go again.

That's what I am thinking.

As if it wasn't bad enough I was crying, once I start telling her what is wrong it will take even longer to calm me down after I am done telling her what is wrong.

I think I am experiencing PTSD.

June 16, 2013

I start seeing my therapist Sal again. My mom thinks it will be best for me to talk to him and tell him what I am feeling, and I don't hesitate to call him, and he says come in to the office and my mom and I go there and I start talking about everything and of course the tears start again.

The first thing I talk about is how people who are supposed to be trained to read results couldn't do their job and my MRI was messed up a whole year ago.

"What do you want to do about this?" Sal asks. "Do you want to sue them? Would that make you feel better?"

"All I want is for them to know what they did wrong and how it affected me, like in my whole life."

"I think she just wants justice," my mom says.

Yeah, I really just want justice but if justice comes with being compensated or being paid off to keep my mouth shut, then that will be a bonus.

That may not be cool, but that's what I am thinking at this point.

After talking to Sal I feel a lot better. So far, he and the doctors at NYU are the only ones I can trust. I am sick of doctors not knowing what to do, being paid for not being able to do their job. I know eventually I will get over it but until then I am going to do my own investigation.

Watch me.

June 19, 2013

I am starting to get less and less pain from my surgery, but after a small seizure in Dr. Sinclair's office in Port Jefferson, which I faked, he put me on another medication. I don't know why I faked a seizure. It was probably the most stupid thing I have ever done in a doctor's office, or anywhere. I just didn't think about it, which was a bad choice on my part.

I went into his office for a checkup and when he left the room I guess I got nervous so I started to rock. I didn't flap my hands, I just stared, and rocked a little, and before I knew it my dad left the room and got the doctor. It was too late. I couldn't just stop because then he would know I was faking, so I just continued. It wasn't long, maybe less than a minute that he was calling my name, and then I snapped out of it.

I didn't provoke the whole thing, but I guess you could say I could have been more in control of what I was doing. I didn't do it just because I wanted to. I guess I got nervous or something.

I didn't want to have a seizure, that's for sure.

I was so used to being surrounded by doctors willing to help me at the drop of a hat that I felt they were my safety net. I was scared to be on my own. I guess I thought I would not be able to function on my own or ever be better again that I figured I might as well keep them on my leash.

Not good.

My thinking is very unnatural at this time.

According to what my mother told me from the lawyer she consulted, unless I was having any health issues from the time of this MRI test we didn't have a case. In my situation, I didn't start having seizures until a few months ago. Between the one year gap of my first test, the tumor must have started growing, and once March came. it was progressively growing, which caused the seizures to start.

This is definitely not an exact science.

June 22, 2013

The fact is, my brain tumor is only responsible for a portion of my anxiety and depression. It has taken me a while to realize this. I tried to blame it on Dr. Iyer in my head because once I was put on Depakote for the seizures, my depression and anxiety did improved but I still am a prodigy of depression and anxiety.

Dr. Iyer never did anything wrong and I have corrected that in my head by forcing it in. But I still can't get over the fact that my tumor was missed.

If only they did their job right, I probably could have gotten this taken care of a year ago.

I keep thinking that.

I still would have probably had to wait to start college, but I could have dodged so many problems with doctors making me worse.

All I can do right now is feel helpless, crying in my bedroom, and feeling like everything is my fault. My mom has looked into two more lawyers, but nothing can be done. I talked to Sal again, and he asked if my parents looked into a lawyer to see if anything could be done and my mom explained to him what both lawyers said.

After that, I broke down crying, I couldn't understand why nothing can be done.

I'm a good person. I wasn't a bad kid. I always did good things in my life, and I could be helped with one small thing.

That's what I thought, and still do.

I keep talking to Sal.

"Remember when you asked me a while ago why I was scared to be home alone, or I always needed something to fill up each hour, or I was depressed for no reason?"

I pointed to the side of my head where I had surgery.

"It's all from this."

Sal smiled, and he tried to help me to understand why nothing could be done, to help me understand that everything was going to turn out fine.

June 30, 2013

At my next therapy session I went in by myself while my dad had a phone interview. Sal and I talked about how I was coping with everything and the first thing I showed him were two letters, one from me that I wrote a month ago after our last appointment, after I started my own investigation.

Hello? I wasn't kidding. I did it.

The first letter was written by me, which I sent to the headquarters of Suffolk County Radiology, which is only 20 minutes from where I live.

Dear Suffolk County Radiology,

I would like to inform you about an unsatisfied patient of yours. I'm Nicole Nagy. About one year ago I had a MRI done in your Smithtown office. Your staff was fine but needless to say your doctors or whoever reads the MRI did a horrible job. A year later, bringing me to March of 2013, I started having seizures, visiting the hospital, and finally had to see a neurologist. His name you don't need to know, but you need to know that after he examined me he urged me to get another MRI done at your office in Smithtown. My mother took me for another MRI with contrast and you wanted to know what showed up.

A TUMOR ON THE RIGHT SIDE OF MY RIGHT TEMPORAL LOBE!

In April 2013 I saw a neurologist and we brought him a copy of the MRI and it was confirmed by him that I had a tumor on the right temporal lobe of my brain. A week later, the neurologist referred me to one of the best surgeons in New York City. The doctor admitted me the same day and told my parents and I that surgery had to be done. It turns out I had a low-grade tumor on the right side of my head.

If you could understand my frustration, why I'm writing to you, maybe you could do your job right. I was away from my home for almost three weeks because of surgery, wires attached to my head, and recovery. It has been five weeks since I have had my surgery and I'm still recovering. I have bad headaches everyday, which sometimes leads me to question if I will ever get better. But anyway, it's not all your fault, so don't worry because the doctors treating me for anxiety and depression should have known or had suggested doing a MRI or something. For years I was told I had learning disabilities, and for years I was treated for anxiety and depression and those medications for anxiety, depression, and concentrating never worked on me because I never had it. What else is sad is all the money my parents wasted on these medicines that never worked and made me worse.

This is where I explain its not all your fault, that I never had anxiety, depression, or a learning disability, and that's because the doctors in the city said it's because I must have had this tumor all along or maybe I was born with it but it grew over time. My doctors in NYC asked me when I was in the hospital if I have ever had a previous MRI.

This is where your mistake comes in. My parents said yes, I had a MRI one year ago at Suffolk County Radiology. The doctors asked if we could get a copy of that MRI so we did that, and when I went for my follow up appointment after my surgery, it turns out the tumor was on your copy of the MRI.

Gee, I wonder, do they like to hide things about people's health or do they just not have qualified doctors working there?

The great thing about this is I'm not expecting anything from you, because of everything I've been through going through outpatient clinics for anxiety, being admitted in hospitals for depression, and feeling hopelessness. I have learned that these experiences have helped me grow and learn who I want to be and where I want to go.

I just want you to know what happened to me so you don't do it to somebody else because I'd hate for somebody to go through what I did. Nobody's life should be turned upside down by a doctor who doesn't know how to read a MRI.

I know you probably won't admit your mistake, but you

should know that as I'm writing this letter to you I'm also working on my own book and this mishap of yours will be in it so don't worry, I won't forget your mistake!

> Sincerely,
>
> Nicole Nagy

The next letter I showed Sal was the reply from their headquarters, which I was surprised I got so quick, but it was not a good surprise, that's for sure. But I wasn't surprised about that, because like I told them, I already knew they would be chickens about taking responsibility for what they screwed up.

Dear Ms. Nagy,

We want to thank you for taking the time to write to us about both your MRI studies at Suffolk County Radiology. We have forwarded your studies for review and education to all of our neuroradiologists.

We wish you all the best in life and health.

> Kind regards,
>
> Suffolk County Radiology

Sal asked me how I felt after writing the letter and if my parents knew I wrote it. I told him they knew. Then he asked me how I felt about the reply.

Getting a reply from them meant bullshit to me.

I didn't say it like that, but you get the idea, because it didn't matter whether Suffolk County Radiology knew about it or not because either way I still had the surgery.

I really wanted justice. I wanted them to know what happened, and that I didn't want the same thing that happened to me to happen to somebody else. I felt let down because I felt like my parents didn't try hard enough—not that I thought they didn't care.

How do I say that stuff?

I wanted to tell Sal that, but if I heard it come out of my mouth I felt I would be so selfish to say something like that. My mom was right, though, because I couldn't harp on it forever and maybe they were trying to protect me from getting hurt.

I guess this is what it's like looking for a lost treasure. I don't have enough to go on, and it's way too hard. Sooner or later, I will get over it and forget it ever happened.

Whenever . . .

July 2013

I reconnected with my old high school guidance counselor and told her about everything that had happened since school. I talked about getting back on my feet, trying to get another job besides working at a bagel store.

I am tired of walking into places and people saying "bagel girl" or when I bring leftovers from the bakery to a nearby church and the people say "bagel girl" again.

There was also the time I was in the hospital to get blood taken and I recognized the nurse and the first thing that came out of her mouth was "bagel store" and that was just so stupid.

I enjoyed working there with the other girls. I just feel that sometimes I have to hide when I go out in public around my town.

That's stupid, too.

Anyway, talking to my old high school guidance counselor was good because she was able to help me get a job working in the high school building for the summer. Most of the time I will be helping Mr. Smith and I also will do small tasks in some of the other offices.

I start next week. I'm still not able to drive for a couple more weeks so my dad will have to go back and forth for me so I can work there.

Thanks, Dad.

July 26, 2013

Will this become a day I'll never forget? Will I lose it? Will I lose my virginity? Don't jump to any conclusions, because life is weird, right?

In the afternoon I saw this movie called *The To Do List* about this quirky girl who makes a list of sexual activities to do before she goes to college. Aubrey Plaza is the actress who plays Brandy Clark in the movie and she is so innocent and doesn't know anything about what I call "the sexually experienced dictionary."

Anyway, the movie was inappropriate and I found it disturbing because there were people humping each other and doing stuff I can't even talk about. After the movie, I felt like I was going to throw up because I was exposed to all this terminology and graphic stuff.

Don't get me wrong. Some parts were funny—very few, but I never would have learned this anywhere else—

not being raised Catholic, that's for sure. Impossible.

There was one scene when one of Brandy's girlfriends was explaining something and Brandy responded "Ew, that's so gross" or something like that, and my boyfriend, Sergio, who was sitting next to me, looks at me and says, "Hey she's just like you."

I think he meant it as a joke, even though he was probably right. I looked at him, like "Shut up! Seriously, that's so rude!"

Okay, this whole thing of me losing it—my virginity——I hate saying that word because it sounds dirty and I don't like that. And I know my dad and his family would be like shocked, or whatever, by the idea of me even using this word, as if it couldn't possibly apply to me, especially when it comes to losing it.

Whatever! I'm not a nun!

So after the movie Sergio and I went back to his house to watch TV. We usually never end up watching anything because we start kissing—a lot, and that's what we did, and when it started to get intense we suddenly stopped and looked at each other.

"Do you wanna try?" Sergio said.

I didn't know what to say. I know it will eventually happen but now? We always talk about it and Sergio was not forcing it on me, but I didn't know what to do.

What? It can't be worse then brain surgery.

I always think that.

One thing led to another and then I stopped Sergio because I just didn't know if this was the day, if this should be the time when everything should change.

Ugh, I feel gross even talking like this.

Sergio never stopped asking me if I was okay. It seemed like it wasn't that big of a deal to him. I mean he's a guy, right? They probably don't show much emotion because they're all like. "I'm a man!"

As I went back to my house a few hours later I was asked myself questions.

Do I feel any different?

Do I look any different?

Am I different, and if I am, how, I mean, why?

My sister saw me walk into the house.

"What's wrong?" she said.

In my head I'm saying, "Holy shit I'm confused, 'cause me and Sergio kind of almost tried to have sex!"

That never came out.

I went upstairs to my room to reflect on what just happened. Here I am, right now, trying to figure this out. I don't remember why we are even considering doing this only two months after me having brain surgery! Losing my virginity is not as scary as the prospect of losing my mind, and I got through that okay, I guess, but this whole thing is too much.

I keep thinking, "Oh my gosh, I'm Brandy Clark!"

How upsetting is that?

That's what I was thinking.

I never told anybody about this except Kaitlyn, and three friends at the bakery. I mean, I don't even know how sex works! I don't! Really! I'm Catholic, remember? It's not that I'm just Catholic, it's that I've never talked about this stuff to my mom or my sister. I feel like it's just assumed that I know about all of this already because of my age, but it's not like I'm comfortable talking about this to anyone in my family.

When I had to go to health class in high school the teacher would let me know in advance if they would be discussing something above my comfort level and I would get a pass and go to the library.

I'm 19, and I still get awkward when I talk about sex.

I don't want to die a virgin—and most important I want it to happen with somebody I love, like Sergio, because I love him, but I don't know when . . .

Tip for young people from someone who doesn't know what she's talking about: wait till you're either in love or when you're really informed because it could hurt like hell—at least that's what it says in the movies. It's probably nothing like they show, so don't get your hopes up. It also isn't something you can plan for, except you can plan *not* to, but who knows how that will work out?

I guess I don't have to do it for a while. I don't know. How do I figure this out?

I didn't have an epiphany today, and I am not exactly on Cloud 9, either.

August 2013

I worked at the high school through the summer and I really enjoyed it! I felt I was learning a lot and was gaining a lot of experience. Some of the days working there I had absolutely nothing to do, but other days I was running around all day.

I felt like I was back in high school, like nothing ever changed.

Towards the end of the month, the director of the program told me that I was one of five people chosen to keep a job throughout the regular school year. I am really happy about that because it is a good job for me where I can't get too overwhelmed. I am also feeling guilty, though, because now on top of going back to school I will also be carrying on three jobs: coaching, school, and the bakery.

Am I guilty, or just freaking out because this is too much?

Next week, I will be starting my first week of school. This year, I will have extra pressure on me because the only way I can keep my scholarship is if I can maintain a B average.

I can't work three jobs while going to school four days a week.

It won't be physically or mentally possible for me.

Why am I even trying to do this?

August 27, 2013

No more bagels!

This is the last weekend before school and my last of my work at the bakery. I really enjoyed working there, but I am tired of being known as the "bagel girl" so when I go out people around town look at me and say, "I know you from somewhere."

I stare at them like no you don't, okay?

I'm always thinking I want to do that, but it's not nice, so I don't.

"Oh, Holbrook Bagels," they'd say, or "Oh, the bagel store," and I'd nod, smile, and walk away fast.

I like all the girls I worked with because they were very nice and Larry, my boss, was the nicest person I ever met, but I quit because my headaches are getting worse and worse and I have to give up one job with school starting because otherwise it will be too much and I don't want my brain to explode.

I did some overtime at the bakery during the week and I remember counting down the days until I had to quit. Now that I'm not there I miss it because I had some much fun there. I was the sales girl because every time Larry came out with something new he would come right to me and say, "Nicole, sell this, or sell that."

"You got it, Larry," and I would sell most of everything we had to people coming into the bakery. Some of the girls laughed and told me I was going to school for the wrong profession, like I should be going to school for a business degree in bagels. I sold a lot because I would use my sarcasm and really get into it, like I was selling cars. People would laugh, smile, and I would be known as the sales woman for the store.

But now—no more bagels!

September 2013

I had to quit coaching soccer and that's killing me. I can't continue while I'm in college because I want to do well and I don't want to have the extra pressure on me. I love coaching, but now after having surgery and recovering slowly I can't coach anyway because my headaches are coming again and coaching makes them worse.

I miss my girls!

That's what I am thinking a lot of times.

My dad is still without a job and each month my paycheck goes away fast. I put half toward my phone and half toward college, so money is tight.

I really love Dowling and I can't see myself at any other college, but when it gets tough I have small breakdowns, which lead to shaking or rocking, like I'm going to have a seizure.

I get PTSD sometimes and it makes me feel all different emotions and sometimes I feel like I can't control it. I get like a small filmstrip in my head. It's like an old movie playing, starting with the doctor's appointment, then finding a tumor, seeing a doctor in the city, finding out I need to be put in the hospital, then no beds available, stuck in the emergency room, crying because some crazy lady is screaming next to me, then another seizure, being in the hospital by myself some nights, having surgery, and so on . . .

Really? *Why did these stupid assholes not tell me I had a tumor a year ago?*

How come nobody can sue them? How come they get away with that? How come nothing was done when Dr. Johnson pressured me to go to dinner with him?

I'm saying that nice, right now, I don't know why, because he sucks, but whatever . . .

I don't understand. None of this is fair. I'm a victim.

I don't want to be that, and I have to stop feeling like this, but whatever . . . *I can't do it that fast so this is how I feel right now.*

That's what happening.

That's the breakdown of my PTSD.

October 20, 2013

Last night before I could go sleep I went to three different websites to look up my former doctor—the pervert—and see if he is still in business. I rated him and left reviews on three different sites saying: I dislike him, he never helped me, and he was treating me for the wrong things.

The whole time I had a tumor in my head, which was causing all my problems, he never looked deeper or bothered to really help me. The wait time to get into his office was often two hours or more.

Not to mention when he tried to get me to go out to dinner with him!

Like I said—pervert.

I really am trying to move forward, but sometimes something rings my memory right back to everything I went through and it puts me in an angry mood and writing a letter, for example, is my way to vent. I know it seems like all I'm doing in just harping on the past, but I'm trying to move forward.

I started school a month ago and so far I am doing well. Sometimes, I daydream in class and I see myself or think like, what if I just have a major seizure right now and drop to the floor and then everybody is standing around me and I'm pronounced dead?

I'm not crazy. I don't know what I am, but I'm not that.

I'm fighting as hard as I can to prove to everybody and myself that I can do this.

I'm going to make it.

That's like a song I'm singing in my thoughts, except this is real for me and I don't always believe it, but when I do accomplish something at school, for example, or I help somebody at work, that is a reassurance for me.

I always tell Sal my therapist about my thinking.

Look where I am now, and where I used to be!

I listen to him as he says, "You're going to have a bright future."

I agree and smile, but inside I feel like it is pressure on me. I want to do great. I want to finish college and become a social worker. Sometimes, I think I'm the one, maybe the only one, who puts too much pressure on me.

Tomorrow I will be 20—whoopee doo.

November 2013

I have a follow up appointment in New York City only this time my aunt isn't coming. It's not her fault that I ended up in the hospital again this past summer, but it's safer for me if she doesn't come. To be honest, it was her fault because she thought I had a seizure and told my doctor. He wanted to make sure I wasn't having seizures, so I ended up in the hospital, and so yeah, she's not coming. I know my aunt was only telling the doctor what she saw, even though it wasn't right, that she was just watching out for me, and I'm much better now.

When I went into the office and my doctor came in, he evaluated me with the usual tests I was familiar with already, only this time I could lift my arms up, push my doctor away, press my fingers together really fast, and bend and flex my feet.

When I arrived back home, I went straight to my work and pushed myself to get as much done as I could get. Whenever I get headaches or migraines they come in different ways, like twitching head pain, pain in the back of my head, pain in the front and back of my head. When they happen, I don't know what to do anymore because I'm loaded on medication.

Aaahhh!

I refuse to give up. I'm going to make it through my first semester back in school and I'm going to work my ass off.

I've started going to "Girls Night" with my friends who I used to work with at the bakery. When I left the house the other night to go out with them my mom asked me where I was going and I replied like this:

"I'm going out to become the normal young woman I was meant to be before I had surgery."

I don't know what that meant, but it sounded good and she laughed and I made a dramatic exit.

At Dowling, I'm in a program called Student Support Services and I am stuck with a woman named Jane, who is an advisor at my college who I meet with each week to talk to and let her know how school is going and if I need help with anything.

I have never been so repulsed by anybody in my entire life.

Every time I meet with her she makes me feel worse and worse about myself.

On Halloween, I brought her one of my research

papers to look over and all she did was bark at me, saying, "Why would you have this here? Why is this there? Does this make sense to you? Read it out loud!"

Beside the fact that she doesn't understand I had freaking brain surgery a few months ago, she always has a nasty attitude and I feel that every time I come to her for help she gets irritated.

After I left her office that day I went to class and for the whole hour and a half I was thinking of different ways to commit suicide. I never felt so close to an idea of hurting myself.

The least painful way to die is the sleeping liquid I sometimes take at night.

I was almost at the point of crying in class, but I was able to keep breathing just enough to keep my cool. When I saw Jane and left her office, I felt even worse.

I feel like a horrible person, like I'm not good enough to achieve anything in college.

When I got home I cried for an hour and smacked my head.

What's wrong with you?

That's what I kept saying to myself.

Sometimes, I don't know how much more I can take.

My mom was holding me in her arms on the couch and she told me there are other options if school is too much. I had my hands over my ears, crying.

I want to go to college! I don't know what else I'd do if I didn't go to school!

I always say I will become a nun or kill myself because I don't want to settle for less.

Why the hell am I still seeing this woman, Jane?

I went to Dr. Miller, who is head of the service, and she told me I could switch to the other lady, Dawn, who is such a sweet person. She goes to church a lot, not like that has anything to do with anything. But I can't switch until next semester, or if I want to see Dawn instead of Jane I have to make arrangements because of my stupid "special" bus, which I take everywhere because I can't drive until I'm cleared from a doctor.

After my meeting with Dr. Miller I cooled off and stopped worrying about Jane. I continue to work my butt off in school, even with migraines every other day. I was enjoying all of my classes and I was interested in everything I was learning. I continued to see Jane once a week, and after I met with Dr. Miller I felt like Jane eased up on me. We actually laughed, and she helped me with stuff, and she was a lot nicer and not as hard on me.

I came to the conclusion that maybe I overreacted, that Jane was pushing me to the best of my ability. I'm in college and much older now and nobody is going to hold my hand. Jane was just saying how it is and I've come to accept that. I take it as motivation to work harder.

I decided I wasn't changing my advisor for next semester because I am able to connect with Jane better and understand where she is coming from. I told my mom that Jane is just doing her job, telling me straight up that this is what I need to do, and how to do things right. I might have thought she was rough at first, but if I didn't have somebody like Jane to remind me how college really is or how to apply myself, I might not be doing as well this semester.

December 2013

I am so relieved the semester is finally over because I worked my butt off and now I am a real college student—again. I should feel tired as hell from pushing myself to the best of my ability.

Over the break, I am spending a lot of time with my family, and I met Lou at his house for lunch. Every time I talk to him he reminds me how much I idolize him, and I want to follow in his footsteps, because Lou is such a good person and he is a great mentor to me.

He told me about his new job, and how he visits children upstate and talks to them and helps them. I never met a person like Lou. After talking to him for just five minutes he gives you the sense of hope that you can accomplish anything.

I'm also entering into a new year by opening up my report card.

Holy shit!

Excuse my language, but holy shit!!!

INTRODUCTION TO ANTHROPOLOGY: B

WORLD RELIGION: B+

SELF & SOCIETY 2: A-

FUNDAMENTALS OF SPEECH: B

I can't believe the grades I got. I had brain surgery like seven months ago and I was able to pull off this great report card!

I should have received an A in speech because I'm freakin Nicole Nagy.

That's what I am feeling because I'm a natural speech giver and my last speech in class was on my brain surgery.

Hello?

Anyway, the first thing I'm going to do is take a picture of my grades and send it to my sister, with a note:

Take that, stupid Suffolk County Radiology!

I say that, even though I don't know how my grades apply to them. Maybe it's to tell them, "See your mistake, and look at me now."

Yeah, that sounds better! This brings me to a new chapter in my life . . .

January 2014

Time flies by quicker than the blink of an eye. In two days I will be going to the city to see my doctor for a check up. But I'm confused. The last two days I haven't had a headache. I cut down one of my medicines on my own, and I think that may have taken away a lot of the head pain I have been experiencing.

I don't want to sound ungrateful, but it's been three full days now, and I don't have much head pain at all, which is weird, and basically I don't like that.

What do you mean, you don't like that?

I'm used to having headaches all the time, so it's not that I miss them, but if nothing is wrong with me, then who am I? I've gone to the hospital so many times that I feel I need to go sometimes because it's what I do.

I told my mom that I get worried if there is nothing wrong or I have no pain. What do I tell the doctor then, if I have no pain? A week ago, I kept saying that when

I get to the doctor I'm going to tell him I'm not leaving until you give me something for my head or fix me.

Maybe I'm just over thinking things.

I think like that a lot—too much—can't stop.

The headaches could come back.

My mom thinks I have to tell Dr. Iyer or talk to Sal. I guess I do, because I get worried so easily that there has to be something wrong with me. If I still have pain then I'll end up in the hospital in the city and they will run tests for a couple of days. I don't know, so I guess I'll wait until I go to the doctor and see what he says.

My mom thinks I feel this way because I've gone to the hospital a lot, and when I told her what I was feeling she got real serious.

"Look at me, look at me," she said.

I looked at her.

"There is nothing wrong with you, and that's a good thing!"

I guess it's a good thing.

This is going to sound very ungrateful, but sometimes I wish I could have had cancer, or my guilty pleasure is that something could happen to me—not death, but enough that I would be in the hospital. I shouldn't say I wish I had cancer because obviously there are people who are suffering from it or who have loved ones suffering from it or who have passed away.

I know that. I'm not stupid.

Maybe I am thinking this way because I don't understand what it feels like, or mainly because it's just the way I feel.

January 27, 2014

I just tried my first alcoholic beverage. I don't mean to sound like an alcoholic, but it was the best thing I have ever tasted! I had an "Adult Root Beer," and if you don't know what that is it's vanilla ice cream, I think, with vodka and some root beer. I didn't get drunk—obviously—but that's because I really can't have alcohol with the medicine I'm on.

But if I could . . .

I was with my family for my mom's birthday and my parents let me try it. When the waitress put the drink in front of me I exchanged looks with my family.

Here goes nothing!

It was really good! It tasted like a root beer float! I started sipping, and my parents got worried, not really, like, they were laughing.

"Oh no, she likes it!"

"Oh gosh, this is bad, ha ha!"

I was only allowed a few small sips because my mom and dad were scared I would have a seizure or something from the alcohol.

At least I can say I finally had a real drink, but if I were to have just straight vodka I don't think I would like it. Before I took a sip, my sister wanted to take a picture and put it on Instagram, I said sure, so she did.

Wait! Don't do that!

That's what I was thinking because I'm going to be a politician, and years from now that could be the picture they (whoever they is) will use against me.

I felt alive, not just because I had a few sips of alcohol, but because I also tried lobster dumplings, and I never ever eat fish. I hate fish. I think its gross, and lobster dumplings might sound gross, but they were great, better than I thought they would be, like chicken salad.

Sometimes you just gotta live a little . . .

February 2014

I recently became a fellow (volunteer) for this organization called Organizing for Action. I heard about it through an email I received from school, and I jumped right on it as soon as I read the details. I took the train to the city all by myself. I almost didn't make it because I had to convince my parents I could go on my own.

The training was at John Jay College of Criminal Justice. I admit, I was very nervous to go by myself, and the cab drive dropped me off four blocks in the opposite direction, so I had to find the place, and then there were a lot of people there.

Long story short, what I thought would be a life-changing program only lasted two weeks for me. When I first left the training, I thought it was amazing. I thought I was supposed to be there, that this was my golden opportunity to start something I'm great at—reaching out to people, advocating for things, and volunteering.

After a few days went by, I was high on life because I thought I had found my calling and I felt nothing can bring me down now!

I boasted to my professors, co-workers, and family.

"Oh this is so great. This is what I'm doing. This is a policy I'm working on."

Yada, yada.

I'm not a really concentrated political person, and before this I'd never followed political news. I don't know how to say it, but I follow *Saturday Night Live* and I vote.

Okay I know it's a privilege to be able to vote.

I can be thinking that, and maybe you are, too, but you should also know about the person you vote for, and other stuff, too.

Before getting involved in a program like OFA I never considered any of this. I didn't really know what political party I was with, and I know that's not the only reason why people vote for the person they vote for, but let me just put it out there.

Anyway, through this program and listening to my professor's banter on how they don't like President Obama and what a mess he is making of this county, I started to take an interest in all of this and my professor's beliefs were maybe getting in my head. In my two weeks of working with OFA, one of the major polices

I was helping to advocate was Obama Care. In class, my professor for global health systems makes me really think and makes me question things.

My point is, from questioning things like Obama Care and other polices I advocated for—ones I didn't really know anything about, by the way—I learned that I didn't like some of the things the President was enacting, but I really liked him and his wife.

I can be such a free thinker now!

I don't identify as a Republican or Democrat. I don't know much about the whole system. I'm still in the early stage of forming my own opinions about things. Basically, in the last couple of weeks I have gained knowledge about policies, but most of it comes from going to college because that is where I learn to question things and understand how much I enjoy learning.

I don't regret volunteering and putting in the time for OFA because it opened up my eyes. Also, it's not like I was doing something I didn't enjoy. It's just that I was advocating for things I didn't really understand at the time, but this experience has given me a better knowledge of things. These people had introduced themselves as a bi-partisan group. Then my professor tells me that the organization's previous name was Organizing for Obama. On top of that, the person in charge of the volunteers from my district told me I was the only one putting in the effort to volunteer and make all these phone calls. That figures, since I'm such a dedicated and hard worker.

Well, they lost me.

That's what I was thinking at first, and then I decided to stop volunteering for them.

Like usual, Dr. Iyer has increased my medicine. I should make another appointment to talk with Sal.

I am never steady. I am always up and down.

I don't know if this is from my surgery or my depression. I mean, come on, with all these meds in my system all these years—okay, not all at once, duh, but still, they've got to be having some weird effects on my body and my brain, I mean, hello?

Every freaking thing you can imagine or can't pronounce— I've been on it.

This list, which, ha ha, I put in alphabetical order just because it keeps me busy for a minute, it includes anti-depressants, anti-convulsants, anxiety this, anxiety that, migraine medication, seizure stuff, and whatever else doctors have felt the need to put me on and I had to take because I just had to.

Abilify

Ambien

Ativan

Botox injections for migraines

Celexa

Concerta

Cymbalta

Depakote

Effexor

Elavil

Fluroset

Inderal

Keppra

Klonopin

Lamictal

Lexipro

Luvox

Maxalt

Neurontin

Nucynta

Pamelor

Paxil

Prozac

Rexulti

Serquol

Steroid shots for migraines

Topamax

Trazodone

Trigger point injections for migraines

Trileptal

Trokendi

Valium

Vilazodone

Wellbutrin

Xanax

Zoloft

Whatever!

I just wonder who I would be without this stuff.

March 2014

Soon it will be a year since I had my brain surgery. I'm still having freaking headaches, nothing helps, and I have more and more appointments each week. Since my dad still isn't working, he has been driving me all over Long Island to doctor's appointments.

He made me laugh in the car because he said we were on a "Stop the Pain" campaign.

When one doctor doesn't have an answer they send me to another.

This just doesn't stop!

In one week, my dad and I have gone to doctors in Commack, Great Neck, Port Jeff, and then two other doctors I see nearby. I would have had seven appointments that week, but I had a bad migraine and drove myself to the hospital on Thursday, missing two appointments for that day, but so what?

Can any doctor figure me out?

April 2014

My dad started working again!

That not only takes pressure off of me, but the rest of my family, too. It's like nothing ever changed!

Even better, I'm no longer dealing with migraines. Now, they're just small headaches, so things are slowly improving. I don't know how this happened, but it did.

Enjoy it while it lasts.

A few days ago, I got accepted into this Washington, DC summer internship program. That's right, you heard it first. I am going to DC this summer for two months and I'm going to help turn this country around!

The only thing that can stop me now is my neurologist, so when I go see him tomorrow I have to ask him and see what he says. I don't think it will be a problem. I haven't had any seizures since before my surgery, and all I have to do is make sure I bring a two-month supply of my medicine. I think it would be a great—no,

EXCELLENT—experience and opportunity for me and I have never traveled anywhere before, especially for two months. I'm so excited.

On the off chance I can't go, of course I'll be crushed, but I always have a back-up plan, which is summer courses and working.

I go to my neurologist with my mom and we tell him I want to attend this program.

He obviously wasn't going to be an ass about it.

"It would be a great opportunity," he said, "and if you really want to go, Nicole . . ."

He went on and on, like whatever . . . I'm going.

I don't think he wanted to be that guy who gets in the middle of a decision that is really up to my parents, because he said it was fine and I have to carry pain medicine in case I get a really bad headache and stuff, but how hard is that to do?

My mom said if I really want to go, maybe I can, which was an amazing start until my dad gets home and they both have to agree, because the fact is, in my situation any parent would be "like hell, no" after going through everything I did and still having headaches.

When my dad got home I overheard him talking to my mom downstairs.

Really? Do they really think I can't hear them or I'm not listening?

I don't know, but I just pretend I'm not, and then my parents come upstairs, and even though I already know the answer one of them comes in anyway and says I should sit down.

"Oh, well, we talked, and . . ."

I think that's what was said, or something like that, and I nodded.

Yeah, or whatever . . .

The only thing next was to get my reimbursement from my school of money I didn't use that school year and little things, like call the insurance company to see if my health care would be good if I went outside of New York, because God forbid if I have to go to a hospital.

God forbid something, okay?

I was excited, knowing I would be staying on campus at American University, one of the best topnotch schools in the country! Away for 2 months every time I thought about it I'd say

Whoa! Away for two months. Bye, Mom. Bye, Dad. See you in two months!

Every time I thought about it, that is what I would say to myself.

But I also had to think about leaving Sergio for two whole months. I guess it would be fine because he went to Brazil once for a whole month in the summer while I was home.

I will miss him a whole lot. He's the love of my life.

I am thinking that, for sure, but I mean, it's Washington freakin' D.C., the most historical, and of course political place, in the country.

I eventually told him I was planning on going, and he was a little upset, but he accepted my choice and he only wants the best for me.

I am gloating to almost everybody about going. I'm trying not to, like I keep planning in my head that what if I meet this person or that person, but I can't help saying something.

But wait. Can I do two whole months away from my family?

I keep thinking that and saying stuff like, "Bye, Mom. I'll see you in two months!" and the more I say it, the more I keep going back and forth, which is what I usually do when I go all OCD on decisions every once in a while. On top of that, I am still having headaches, even if they are not major, but they are every day. Will the heat really be okay for my head?

The next day at school, I tell Jane the good news and she gives me a huge hug.

"I knew you would get it!"

I talk to her about the pros and cons of me going away for two months.

Before I submit an application to the program Jane helps me sign up for summer courses, in case things don't work out exactly like I think they can.

I don't know. I don't know.

I keep OCDing in my head to the point where Jane tells me she won't withdraw me from the summer classes until I make a down payment for the internship in D.C.

Why is choosing stuff so hard?

July 2014

In the end, Jane's idea of signing me up for summer school turned out to be a good idea because I decided not to go. I think it was best, because I probably wouldn't have been able to adjust to living so far away for that long without my parents and everything else that is familiar.

Not yet!

Plus, I can keep working at the school through the summer and make money!

From there on, I just kept a positive mind. Sure, I was disappointed, and felt I had to explain myself to people after I told them the first news that I got into this program. It was my last day working at the high school. I was excited because I could just work one job and relax before going back to school.

I was especially grateful because I would no longer have to see Mr. Smith. I did a lot of crap for Mr. Smith, and now I realize that. Teachers and staff that knew me would joke around and say he was overworking me or that I was his slave.

Maybe they are right.

One day, I was in front of the school planting trees and flowers under the digital board in front of the school, which kinda pissed me off at the time because after 20 minutes out there I was wondering what was going on.

Shouldn't the janitor or maintenance guy be doing this?

Really, that's what I was thinking, which was the right thought to be having.

Or the time I was carrying Christmas trees from one side of the school to the front and bringing them up into the attic above the auditorium with some of Mr. Smith's in-school suspension kids. At the time, I just smiled and shrugged it off because I thought Mr. Smith and me were buddies. I was a hard worker and I always wanted to keep busy. But now that I think about it, I am shaking my head because it looks like a different story.

I am pretty sure I was his lackey.

We worked closely together, so it was just natural that he gave me his phone number, which I guess was for work purposes. But then inappropriate messages started after I sent him a picture of my cat by accident in a group message I sent to my friends. The photo was me holding my new kitten, Frankie, and in a private message he replied "Lucky Kitty."

Creepy or okay?

Sometimes, it was normal conversations and I didn't think anything of it, but on other days I received weird texts from him. I'd ignore it, or pretend I didn't get it when I went into work. I guess I wasn't completely innocent, but I thought it was normal because I knew him for such a long time and he was very nice to me.

I was a kid!

I thought it was very generous of him to get me a job two months after having brain surgery.

This is the last conversation I had with him, which is what led me to tell my parents.

7/24/2014

Want to go boating?

You have a boat?

Yes

When?

Any afternoon next week

Call me

Okay I'll let you know when I'm off! Sounds fun!

Can you call me?

Yeah next Tuesday is probably good for me!

Perfect about 1 the boat is in east Islip but I can meet you somewhere and drive you to the boat

Okay can I bring Sergio?

Is that what you want to do

I would like to, is that alright with you?

I would like spending time with you but will do anything you want

I would feel more comfortable if he came, if that's okay

Ok 1 o'clock you and Sergio

we can try a little fishing then try beach

Okay! I'll bring lunch! Just send me the address

K I will text you directions tomorrow

Okay sounds good!

Can we do 2 I forgt I have a doctors appointment?

Call me when you can if Tuesday is not good we can try another day

Okay I call you Monday?

Call me now

I'm kinda tired I just got home, I'll call you tomorrow afternoon

K

After this, I blocked and deleted Mr. Smith's number. Sergio knew about it, but I always wanted to see the best in people so I just kept my distance and limited my conversations with him outside of work. Occasionally, I would go back to the school to visit, just to see some of the staff I worked closely with in the attendance office because they were such sweethearts to me.

Sometimes, they'd say "Oh, Nicole, hey, did you see your buddy?"

They were referring of course to Mr. Smith, but I would be nonchalant and laugh.

"No, I didn't get around to it."

I wasn't mad at him. I didn't hate him, but I just needed to distance myself from him, because maybe one adult perv in my life was already enough.

How many pervs does it take before you just say "enough!"

August 2014

I believe things happen for a reason, and in a positive way things end up working out for me.

I recently won a leadership scholarship from Dowling! As soon as I read the email I called by mom.

"I still got it!"

And in the fall semester I am going to be the new president—yes I said president—of the Humanitarian Club. It was going to happen sooner or later.

Nicole Nagy: President of the Humanitarian Club.

It has a nice ring to it!

As the summer progressed, I was already into my second course learning about long-term health care! Up to this point, my idea of nursing facilities was smelly, depressing, and dirty. My own thoughts and opinions changed completely by the end of the course. I learned directly from the source because my professor is a former supervisor of a nursing facility. He taught us all the ins and outs, from cleaning services to Medicaid and Medicare. I interviewed staff and residents at a nearby nursing facility and conducted a full report.

This summer I felt pretty good. I lowered my seizure medication each week. I've been jobless, but keeping busy. It sounds great, but when I received my monthly bill from Dowling, that changed really quick because it turns out that the school is taking my grant away because my parents' income has increased. When my dad got a new job the salary was lower than his old job where he got laid off but combined with my mom's income it's still was too high for me to hold on to my grant. Instead of paying $17,000 dollars in tuition, now we—my parents, mostly—have to pay $24,000. Alisa, my sister, is already paying over a thousand dollars a month and she keeps warning me to leave and says it's not worth it.

I have to make the hardest decision of my life.

That is, in my 20 years I've been on this earth.

In the next two weeks I will resign as a Dowling student and became a full-time student at Suffolk Community College.

September 20, 2014

Let's just get it out there. Suffolk is nothing compared to Dowling. Suffolk is a large fish bowl and the professors and staff are sharks! All the fish (students) and I are just swimming around, doing our own thing. But when I need help, let's just say some of the sharks have no idea or are just concerned about themselves. At Dowling, everybody cares, from the professors to the faculty. They truly help you succeed.

The first two weeks of school have been rough. I dropped a philosophy class because it was a different language to me and every time I get help I still leave confused. I'm taking remedial math because my brain is dysfunctional when it comes to numbers and stuff.

For the past few days coming home from school I have banged my head multiple times against my math textbook, squeezing my face. I thought I was going to give myself a concussion because I was really hitting my head hard. Not to mention, I was standing in the kitchen with a long knife to my head, like really, I was kind of poking the knife into the right side of my head, a little bit, but still. My mom was on the computer at the kitchen table and didn't notice. I put the knife back and went over to her and asked her if she saw what I did and she said no. I said I was glad, but then I told her what I did and she made me sit down at the table.

"Why would you do that?" she said.

My fists were clenched. I was a mess. All I wanted to do was die and never wake up again. I'm not sure if it was the math class getting to me because I couldn't understand, or something else.

If I can't pass this stupid math it's going to hold be back becoming a social worker.

I kept thinking that the first two weeks of school.

Seriously though, I won't even need math in my profession it's so frustrating because people have to take classes they won't ever use in the real world—not all, just some.

September 22, 2014

I called my mom on the way home from school and said I want to drive into a pole and never wake up. I keep getting tantrums from school. I never would feel like this if I were at Dowling because I would be getting the help I deserve and need.

Later, I overheard my mom talking to my dad, saying Suffolk is ridiculous, that they are a bunch of assholes there because they don't help me or do anything.

It kind of made me laugh and cry at the same time.

"Well, the amount you pay for school amounts to the quality of education you receive."

That's what I told them.

Therefore, that's Suffolk for you!

My mom said to me that if I truly wanna go back to Dowling I can go right ahead, but it mean I will have a large bill, like with a student loan.

"I think you will succeed, Nicole."

She said that, which was good.

Maybe I will just stay here because I only have a few more requirements to fulfill to transfer to Stony Brook, which is where I want to go to become a social worker, anyway. I need a math tutor, a therapist, and I don't know what else, but probably something. I have to see Dr. Iyer now to tell her what's going because I have been banging my head against my books and squeezing my face.

"How to do you expect to become a social worker if you can't even control your own frustration?" my mom keeps saying.

She's right, okay?

I'm going to be helping people control stuff like that so I have to get together.

October 21, 2014

It's been a few weeks but here I am—alive and doing better. I can't believe I finally made it to 21 years old. Pardon my French, as they say, but "Holy fuckin shit!"

Really, holy shit! Holy shit! Holy shit!

I keep saying that to myself because I never thought I would make it this far! I always assumed I was going to die before the age of 21. It's kind of overwhelming, though, now that I am, and I'm starting to feel anxious. I don't know why I'm so anxious because this is a cool milestone for me and I should be happy!

It's just that I really didn't think I was going to make it this far—like for years I always couldn't imagine what my future would be like, or what I was going to do with myself, if that makes any sense. I guess part of the reason I felt this way for so long is because of the lesion in my brain and I guess I got used to feeling like that and it became normal for me.

Feeling all weird and bad becomes normal and that's messed up. It really is.

I've been thinking that for a long time, I guess.

Anyway, I'm in my second month at Suffolk Community College and I hate it here. I'm sure other people like it but not me. I hate it here. It's a joke. First of all, I feel like I'm back in high school. Second, none of my professors are making an impact on me. Third, I'm not getting any help from the school.

Three big reasons for it to suck!

December 8, 2014, 9:27 a.m.

The last few days, I have been getting tight fisted and epileptic. I notice it always happens toward the end of the night. My mom thinks it's because I'm working too much. But how else can I do good in school?

There is always part of me that wishes something bad would happen to me. That's always been my guilty pleasure.

I think I am part psychotic.

I don't know why, when half the time I'm positive and I can't wait for the future because I think I am going to be very successful.

Maybe this psychotic stuff is from my brain surgery.

I think my brain surgeon misconnected some wires during my surgery. Maybe my period is making me like this. It usually does, or maybe it's because I'm reading this new book, *Brain on Fire*.

December 8, 2014, 4:41 p.m.

I just got home from work and I wanna die. On the drive home I wanted to crash my car into something. I wanted to be in the ambulance, speeding down the road . . .

I want out.

If I am thinking this, how come I can't kill myself? Is it because I'm Catholic?

How much more can I take till it's too much?

December 24, 2014

Fast forward to Christmas Eve and my report card:

PSYCHOLOGY — A

The professor is a depressive and I kinda related to her so I spoke up a lot and shared my thoughts. She didn't do anything, so easy grade.

ENGLISH — B

I expected this because the professor was way better than the usual Suffolk quality and should be teaching at Yale or something. She is the most decent professor I've had so far.

REMEDIAL MATH — R

It just says R, which I'm assuming means retake.

There is absolutely no way I'm taking this class over because the professor sucked.

I am thinking this right now, remembering exactly what the stupid rating said on ratemyprofessor.com, that the professor was good. He sucked! I ended up getting a tutor and cheating the whole course and final, and wait. Here's what R means.

I failed?

Seriously, what the fuck?!

This was the first time I actually started understanding math, thanks to the tutor my mom hired, and I was getting good grades on the quizzes and tests and doing all the homework. I wasn't really cheating. I just had help from this good tutor, so I didn't do it all by myself, but I did the quizzes and tests myself and my tutor helped me with my homework, but so what?

Whatever . . .

This has ruined my whole day. I don't even feel like going to work now.

I'm a stupid-ass. I hate myself. I wish I were dead. Please give me a tumor, God so I die.

Here come those thoughts, etc., etc. etc.

I ended up going to work anyway, feeling like crap. I can always put up an invisible shield of how I feel and nobody can ever figure what's wrong with me, like I have a really good poker face. I'm good in those ways.

I can even fool myself.

I ended up getting home early Christmas Eve and I am home alone. Usually, my family and I would be opening gifts because the next day my mom will be working, but this time my family is at church with my grandma.

I don't want to face the world. I was really depressed so I got impulsive and I took eight melatonin pills, and left a note.

Yes, I tried to commit suicide but it was unsuccessful.

That's why melatonin is the safest sleeping medicine because you take only one and you fall asleep in an hour. Try and take eight and you're way drowsy, but that's it. I thought I figured out the best way to end it and it would make a great story

BREAKING NEWS:

CHRISTMAS MORNING!

FAMILY WAKES UP TO FIND THEIR 21-YEAR OLD DAUGHTER DEAD.

All I wanted to do was go peacefully.

I was tired in a depressive way and I didn't want to be bothered anymore. When my parents got home I was in my room, tossing and turning because the stupid melatonin didn't even make me sleepy. I heard my mom calling my name. I guess she got the note! She came rushing into my room, shaking me, as I tried to pretend I was sleeping.

What? What? I'm trying to sleep!

Then the light came on. It was like a family intervention with my mom asking me "What did you take, Nicole?" and I didn't want to answer because it was so stupid.

At this point, I think I would have qualified for a *60 Minutes* special on CBS or a medical study for mental illness.

The list of medications I've tried is unreal . . .

December 25, 2014, 8:30 a.m.

My suicide was unsuccessful. I'm still here—probably because I took natural sleeping pills.

Idiot.

I really don't think I passed my stupid ass remedial math class.

WTF?

Yesterday after work, I was really contemplating driving into a pole or a tree, thinking I was such a stupid-ass, piece of shit.

You stupid-ass piece of shit!

If I had a tumor and only a few months to live I'd be so happy right now. I'd be okay with it. I am praying to God to let that happen, or maybe something could go wrong with my recent MRI, but I got zero problems there and I don't know what to do.

I hate my life and I wish I were dead.

January 13, 2015

All I wanted to do is exercise, but I got tight—in my head and I couldn't.

Was it from small talk?

Was it from making plans around my school schedule?

Was it seeing my boyfriend . . . or depression—again?

I'm so tired of guessing why I feel like this.

My head just met a kitchen cabinet door, and then a book called *40 Days to a Healthier Life*, and then a metal water canteen.

It doesn't hurt—my head.

I guess I will feel the pain in the morning.

I called Dr. Iyer. God bless this woman for being the best doctor I've ever had who is able to keep up with me (almost) and have patience. I take half a Zoloft in the morning and half a Klonopin at night with my Zoloft.

My mindfulness is making me be acceptable—if I were a vegetable.

January 26, 2015

I envy people that took their own lives because they had the courage to do the one thing I can't succeed at. I wish I was on death row or that woman who moved to Kentucky or some creepy place because she had brain cancer and she gave consent to the doctors to inject her with something and she could go peacefully.

My thoughts are my deadliest weapons.

I know that and should not think it, but it's the truth, so I am thinking it all the time, whether I like it or not.

I should have ended up in the ER last night for taking either three Klonopin or I think Nuycentas, I don't know for sure, but I got out of it. Ever since I started this new medicine I've been having dreams of being chased and I've been waking up in a pissy mood.

I don't give a flying fuck about myself.

I look forward to the day I can finally rest in peace.

Amen.

February 2015

The world tipped in my favor—temporarily, at least. I was able to get through the next math course, even though I failed remedial math. One of the counselors was able to remove the R from my record because I passed the next level math.

At this point, I do not hate Suffolk as much as I used to, but I'm not in love with it, either. It's kind of on probation. It's like a gas station or pit stop—fill up on the bullshit courses you need and head to your next destination, in this case for me, Stony Brook.

For the spring semester at Suffolk I am registered for Statistics, U.S. History and Spanish. History and Spanish are a breeze so far but Stats is the most difficult I ever had. I have a tutor, and on top of that I am staying after class with the professor every single day.

I was also seeing a therapist at school with a really complicated last name so I called her Dr. V. She's a nice lady, but things have not worked out between us. I could tell early on I was too much for her.

"It's okay," I told my mom. "I can admire somebody who walks away from a challenge, in this case me!"

My mom laughed.

Although things didn't work out with Dr.V., I learned some coping skills from her. Each time I saw her I'd hand in a writing log and we'd talk about it, but I think she was afraid I might commit suicide, and from a doctors perspective they don't want to be held responsible.

"Hello, Mr. and Mrs. Nagy? Hi, this is Dr. V., and I'm really sorry, your daughter finally did it, but it's not my fault."

Can you imagine?

Dr. V. told me that she didn't want me to think I was being "abandoned" but really that meant something else and I knew that.

If anything happens to you I don't want to be sued.

That's what I was thinking she was thinking because it's true.

March 2015

I'm not doing too well right now. I'm starting to go off my Keppra and my beloved Zoloft that I have been on for years because it has stopped working.

I am a mess.

I am banging my head again, writing the most terrible things on my writing log, which I am still doing, even though I don't see Dr. V. anymore. She was really worried and kept having me sign a contract, saying I wasn't going to harm myself. During our time when I saw her, I signed three of them.

Eventually, I called Dr. Iyer and soon enough I was at St. Catherine's Hospital in Smithtown. My time there wasn't bad because it is the cleanest place I've ever been. The other people weren't bad at all and everybody seems to be functioning well. They probably just need their meds adjusted.

I ended up leaving after two days and started

Depakote, which turned out to be really good for me! I look back now and I realize the people I've come across in these different hospitals aren't crazy. They were not mentally retarded or anything, either.

We just have psychological obstacles we are dealing with. Nobody on psych wards, or in psychiatric hospitals, asks to be there. We just need assistance, whether it's with medication or in therapy groups.

We're all the same. I mean you and me.

We're not un-human, us "crazies."

Everybody has their own issues, right?

June 2015

After those two days in the hospital I went back to Suffolk to finish the spring semester. My History professor made me laugh. My Spanish professor was good, too and I went for a lot of extra help. I asked my grandma for help with homework because she speaks Spanish! The roughest class is Stats, especially for a useless math person like me, and I know I will never use it again, or probably not.

Never!

I had a tutor and my professor helped me but I always felt like a two-year old, needing every little thing to be explained.

Why? Why? Why?

Little kids ask that about everything and I wanted to do that, too,

I explained to my teacher that I couldn't break stuff down very easily and that my surgery definitely played a part in that.

That's not an excuse, I mean it is, but it's a real one.

Fortunately, my teacher saw all the time I was putting into the class and just barely passing because during every test I sat with her in her office and she pushed information out of my head that I didn't even know I remembered. I ended up with a C and thanked her from the bottom of my heart in a nice letter I wrote and I left flowers on her desk.

I got a B+ in History and a B in Spanish.

Yes!

The hard work drove me crazy but I'm done.

August 2015

I had to finish a requirement of Biology 101 this summer. I walked in thinking it was going to be just remembering facts and definitions, but I was completely wrong! I ended up getting a tutor because it was another one of those difficult subjects that my brain just can't process.

My mom hired a tutor from the same place we got my math tutor, but he was definitely not as good at all. I don't think much of this guy. For example, when I'd ask him a question he'd say, "Uh, I'm pretty sure its this, yeah," and when I would refer to something in class, he'd say something like "I think he means this, or I think that's what it means, right?"

You're asking me?

I would be thinking that all the time, like, really?

You don't know, but you think?

Should I have congratulated him because he could think? Oh, please! I wanted to say stuff to him like "My mom isn't paying you to think. She's paying you to know!"

She's paying you to help me, you idiot!

I wanted to say that all the time to my tutor, and that should be the last thing you ever want to say because that person *is* helping you.

What a butthead.

It's okay, because in any situation I end up having to rely on myself and from ending with a D+ in the class I convinced my professor to give me a C.

August 15, 2015

I received my acceptance letter from Stony Brook University!

I was sitting in Island Empañada, a little Mexican restaurant, at the time and heard my email go off so I glanced at it and saw who it was from and the subject title was "Regarding your application" and oh my God—

I was accepted!!!

I stopped stuffing my face with rice and beans long enough to said out loud, "Oh my God" and I think I said it pretty loud and I cried a little because the workers looked at me, but I was like, "Eh, I don't give a shit right now, okay?"

My dream just came true!

It was like a scene in a comedy movie: I was the heifer, eating fast food by myself, crying like I just got dumped by somebody. Except I was a living commercial for something amazing, and I didn't care who else knew it because I did, and that was too good to be true, but it *was* true and that made it even better.

The first person I called was the woman who gave me life—my mother. She was freaking out as much as me. Next, Sergio, and then Mr. Medina, and my friend, Ms. Fassano, who is like my third grandma from working at the high school. She said, "Oh, honey, I told you you'd do it, see God is good and you're going to be amazing." She asked me a million questions at once!

I was just so happy, and not to be conceited, *but I deserved this!*

Not that it even had anything to do with all the trials and tribulations I had experienced, but I worked myself through school, going full-time right after my surgery and I worked all those jobs. I pushed myself through homework, reading, and tests while having migraines. Anybody who knows me and knows everything I've been through knows I deserve this and this is all I ever wanted—an actual start at a social work career! I will definitely get that at Stony Brook because I can finish my Bachelors there and then do my Masters.

Oh my God! Oh my God! Oh my God!

The rest of the day I was high as a cloud, not in a stoner way, but in a happy way. Nothing can bother me today and nobody can take away this true bliss because this is my path and I am going to continue to see it through.

August 25, 2015

I've continued working through the summer at Victoria's Secret, hanging out with Sergio, friends, and trying to take it easy. I've never been one to take it easy though, and I am never able to give myself a break. I don't know if its because of all the issues I have or because I never accept anything less of myself and this is the drive that keeps pushing me, but somehow usually everything works out.

I wish I would remember that when I'm freaking out.

Getting into Stony Brook has definitely made me feel more confident and scholarly, I guess you could say. When I'm not working I've visited the school to get familiar with the classrooms and the campus. All of my classes are going to be in the hospital, which is thrilling. Stony Brook Hospital has a school known as the Health Science Center, and that's where all the med students, nursing, physical therapy, and social work students go.

I toured the building a few times and other places on campus, like the writing center and disability services.

There are a lot of international students, mostly in my building, like Chinese, Korean, and Indian people, and my dad works a lot with them.

Anyway, a week or two before school, I naturally started freaking out, having high anxiety, and whatever. I started seeing a therapist named Nikki who is helpful keeping me stable. I still have Dr. Iyer, but Nikki is a social worker, like my last therapist Sal, who ditched me, I guess, because he just stopped returning my calls. Nikki is much better because she is helping me get to a better place where I no longer hit my head against things.

It's nice to not be doing that.

December 2015

I don't know how I made it this far.

I didn't know if I was going to be able to handle Stony Brook. The first month of school felt like learning to swim for the first time, and I was being tested in a cold pool. I had nice professors, and a lot of things we talked about were repetitive, for example, racism issues, homeless issues, and a lot of social injustice issues. We had many readings assigned for each class, like 20 pages at least for one or two classes, which I didn't mind reading until the migraines started to come back.

If I read too much, I get tension between my eyes, and if I over-work my brain I get pain in my forehead.

Sometimes it's too easy to over-work my brain!

I think this because it's true, not just a jokey thing to say, because I am always rubbing my head in class and rubbing my eyes. It can be torture.

I became miserable during the semester because

the migraines and tension in my head was making me depressed and not able to concentrate. I met with my advisor in disability services and expressed my anxiety about school, my migraines, and stress.

I'm in over my head here.

That's what I thought, that I had gotten in over my head with school and I kept hearing my mom's voice in my head, saying, "If its too much for you there are other options," which meant if I couldn't handle school I could quit and do something else.

No!

I would never let that happen because like I always say, I will never accept anything less of myself. I actually always say that.

I will never accept anything less of myself.

See? I just said it.

I ended up getting my textbooks on audio and listening to the chapters and not pushing myself too much. This helped the migraines and all the tension in my head.

It took a month or so to adjust to Stony Brook and one attempted suicide with Nyquil for me to stop pushing myself so much that I was too overworked.

This happened in the middle of October. I was in a CVS parking lot in Holbrook with a bottle of Nyquil, and honestly I was ready.

It was so easy.

All I did was get Nyquil and the lady didn't even ask me anything or notice I looked severely depressed. All she said was, "feel better," like she assumed I had a cold in the middle of a beautiful fall day.

Really, lady? You're just going to let me die?

I didn't want to feel the pain anymore—the headaches, the stress, and the depression. In that moment, I had no regard for my actions or what effect it would have on my family, or Sergio. I never told him what happened after that night. Only my family knew.

By going through with it I'd be giving up all the hard work that had gotten me into Stony Brook, but in that moment I simply didn't care.

When those moments hit, it's not logical, or anything like that.

I felt that by going out this way I could avoid saying life was too hard for me or that I could not handle Stony Brook. Plus, I wouldn't have to go through filling out all the stupid paperwork of withdrawing from school.

Like I said, it's not a logical thing.

I only drank half the bottle, but it was still dangerous. It even says so on the package, like don't drink all of this because it can kill you, or something like that. I was angry that it didn't kill me. It felt like I had failed again, that I couldn't even kill myself right.

After that, my medicine was adjusted again and I told

Nikki what led me to that moment. She tried to put this idea in my head, that since my brain surgery had taken away some of my fears, this can also put me as risk to attempt suicide, so I have to be careful. This is because of the tissue that was taken out on the right side of my head, which controls fear and stuff, so this has been making me less fearful of things.

Maybe you should be more afraid of dying, hello?

I've always been a risk taker, but I guess after my surgery, and on top of having a chemical imbalance, this puts me at risk for attempting suicide.

I think.

Nikki helped me understand my own thoughts so that I can kinda understand my own thinking every once in a while.

Imagine that. I can understand myself!

Maintaining those sessions with Nikki and my new medication helped me feel better so I could get through my first semester at Stony Brook. It took me some time before I realized that Nikki was right. I didn't have to read every single thing in my classes because a lot of it was repetitive and the discussions in class already made sense to me so if I could stay engaged in class I would be cool. Nikki got her bachelor's at Stony Brook!

How did I not end up in the hospital?

I probably just talked my way out of it, as usual.

During mid-term exams, I was still struggling to grasp the concepts, even though I engaged in class and knew everything that was going on. It's just that when it came to taking tests it was difficult for me. I told my professors my concerns and they agreed with me. They said I was participating well and that the tests were my biggest struggle.

I kept trying.

Luckily, when I got back a D or a C- my professors provided extra credit assignments, which helped me. Overall I started feeling more confident and I was doing the most I could to keep up in class. I enjoy learning about these issues in class because I feel like I was learning life lessons, which changed my outlook on society.

Then finals came and I didn't think twice.

I can only do the best I can.

That's what I was thinking all the way through, and usually that is easier said than done but this time I actually stuck to this saying and prospered.

I just received my grades and I am fucking amazed (sorry for my language).

HUMAN BEHAVIOR 1— B

RESEARCH IN SOCIAL WORK — C+

POLITICAL ECONOMY — B

CONTEMPORARY SOCIAL JUSTICE ISSUES — B

SOCIAL WORK POLICY — B+

How about that, ladies and gentleman?

I basically want to cry inside but I feel too good for that now. Each grade feels like a ten- pound weight being lifted off my body, since I've been waiting anxiously for each one.

As I start winter break, I am worried about how I often find it often difficult to keep myself occupied. I always want to relax, but I never give myself the opportunity because I always like keeping busy.

Not that keeping busy is a bad thing.

I am getting to the point of OCDing, like the time before I knew I had a tumor in my head and I was scared of having nothing to do. Luckily, I still have a lot of hours working at Victoria's Secret at the mall, which is a blessing and a nightmare.

While working on and off during the break I will watch a lot of movies on Netflix about people with mental illnesses and although it gets depressing at some points I also find the stories to be inspirational.

I already watched *I'm Not Crazy* with Brittany Snow and Jennifer Hudson and *Veronika Decides to Die.* I told my mom and she asks me why I am watching these.

Why do you watch this stuff? It's gonna make you more depressed!

These movies did make me feel upset for a minute or two, but I feel like I can relate to them and also experience what other people go through. I don't expect my mom or dad to actually understand this completely because they're not the ones depressed and stuff, which is good, and even though I know they love me so much they still can't really get it, but I do.

February 2016

I finally started second semester and was really getting the gist of it. I had the same professors, which I like, and kept volunteering, which has helped me to feel like my old self again. I gained many new friends doing this.

In March, I volunteered with a group in Nashville, Tennessee. It was the best experience. I met the most amazing, down to earth people, and I learned so much about agriculture from working with a food bank.

This trip brought me out of my comfort zone.

When we came back, I quit working at Victoria's Secret. At first, I enjoyed it, but after a dozen nasty encounters with customers, I wanted to kill myself—and them. I know I am not supposed to say something like that, but I'm fine with it. I enjoyed most of the people I worked with, but I did not like the managers. Two of them were okay, but . . . whatever.

The customers were horrible.

Although I had a gift for getting people to open up store credit cards, I think retail is the worst job anybody could have.

I am better than this place and need to find a job where I can excel and use my natural abilities for helping people.

That's what I was thinking while I worked there, and it's not like I am saying I am better than people, I just think I have talents to be used somewhere better. So I started subbing at a special needs school.

Second semester is going well but one class is killing me: Statistics for Social Workers.

I am never going to use statistics—everrrr!

I'll make sure of it! I am not going to be a researcher. I am going to change lives and stats do not make sense to me. I've been down this road before, but everybody is hung up on statistics.

I have to stop engaging in destructive behavior.

I know this is going to sound so stupid, but I tried to commit suicide again. Telling this to the nurse I was thinking, "Really? I tried to kill myself over this?"

It was during my stats class and we were receiving our midterms back and I got a 29. Needless to say, I failed. A girl behind me complained that she got a fuckin 90-something and she was upset that she didn't get a higher grade. Another kid said, "Whoa, I'm so surprised, I did better than I thought."

I hate when people do that.

It's like, seriously, you got a fucking A so what more do you want?

I want to punch those people in the face.

Generally, as long as I get at least a B I'm a happy person and my parents aren't the kind of parents that expect so much out of me when it comes to grades. They say as long as I pass that's all that matters. I have nothing to prove expect being a hard worker.

After that, the Professor went on with the class and I shut down, like when a car breaks down and it doesn't move, and you can't restart it, and then smoke starts.

I was a broken down car.

That's what I was thinking, sitting there with my 29. I bet there was smoke coming out of my ears. I didn't talk for the first two hours of class, and I wasn't moving.

It got worse.

People started to notice because I was having attitudes in my head toward people in the class, like I was hitting them in my mind, and that must've been showing on my face. I was not doing it on purpose, but I couldn't control myself. I had to get home before something bad happened. I left early from class and emailed my professor, saying I had to leave because I felt so and so and needed help.

Luckily, I had the therapist that day so I drove right

over to Nikki's house. I felt like a ticking time bomb, that at any moment as I was driving I would hit a wall, or another car, or somebody would hit me.

I arrived at her house and that was it. I put the car in park, with the engine running, and my Adele CD on. I wrote a note on a piece of notebook paper.

I apologize to my family and my boyfriend Sergio,
but I can't go on like this anymore.
I no longer want to feel ashamed of myself.
I am tired, and I can't take it anymore.

I forget the rest, but you get the idea. It was ten minutes after my appointment was supposed to start and after laying down on the car seat, balling my eyes out, I turned off the car, and walked into her office.

I don't know what made me change my mind.

I don't know what I was thinking, except maybe it was God forcing me out of my car.

I walked into her office like I just saw a ghost. I was still crying and she called out my name and saw my eyes and she gave me a hug.

"What's wrong?"

I told her everything, and she said she had a feeling something was wrong because I came in late.

"You know I would have saved you, right?"

I heard what Nikki said, but I wasn't really there, either, like I didn't know anything about being saved, by anybody, like, why?

At that moment, I was ready to go.

I wasn't thinking about what would happen after. I just didn't want to be angry at myself any longer. I didn't want to bang my head anymore.

Nikki and I called my mom at work and Nikki suggested I should go to the hospital. She ended up driving me to Mather Hospital because it was right by her office.

My therapist is driving me to the emergency room in an orange Mustang.

I kept thinking it was a funny situation, but when I arrived it stopped being funny.

I was put in a small room the size of a walk-in closet. Nikki stayed with me until my parents arrived.

The male nurse asked me why I tried to commit suicide.

"Statistics."

In my mind, I thought did I really just say that? Is that why I'm here? I tried to kill myself over stupid math?

Whatever it was, it doesn't change the fact I tried to commit suicide again.

I wanted help, but if it meant I was going to be taken out of school I didn't want it now. I was almost done and this weekend was Easter and I was planning to go to my cousin Cyrena's house and I wanted to play with my little cousins.

I told Nikki the stuff I was looking forward to and she said if I convinced the doctor of that maybe I wouldn't get committed—or admitted. But if I did get admitted, that would be good for me because they could help me get better and monitor me on different medicine.

This all sounded good to me but I didn't want to miss school. I don't know why my interests changed so quickly from wanting to die, then not dying, and wanting to finish the semester at school. Maybe it was because I was unsuccessful and needed something else to focus on, or to be successful at, in this case, school.

If you don't succeed, try and try again, but I would not try again with suicide.

I was getting twisted in my head, thinking about this, but I just meant that I would try and try again to better myself and continue school. I had to convince the doctor about that.

Phew!

I was sent home that evening, somewhat relieved.

I felt like a magician.

I can cast a spell on my mind or on others to assume I'm not depressed or suicidal. Maybe that makes me a manipulator, or I'm getting stuck in my own head.

That's the one thing about mental illness—you never know if the impulsive thoughts in your head are from your illness or it's your mind being creative—at least that's what I think.

I ended up going back to Dr. Iyer after my trip to Mather.

My brain is sort of being operated on again, like they want to see what these new medications will do, but instead of physical reactions they are trying to fix me mentally.

I'm not saying I need fixing, but I think we can agree that I could use a tune up!

Now that I am done with school, I am trying to force myself to relax, and at times it is somewhat difficult, but I am trying to make it work, especially now that I am being ditched again by my new therapist—not really new, because I've been with her, I think for a year, and she's not really ditching me—she's moving. We had a good run together, but I feel like therapists nowadays are like new sunglasses. They're nice, usually very good to you, but eventually, like all the rest, they don't last very long and you end up getting a new or better pair the next month. Sometimes they break, or they just don't do it for you anymore—anyway you get the idea.

Nikki gave me a referral for somebody she said is like her and would be a perfect fit for me, but she is a little older. Age isn't the problem. I just don't know if I will contact her. Do I really wanna go through the whole process of get to know someone again and telling her my problems and then five or six months later find out she is retiring or moving?

What am I getting out of all this?

July 2016

I can't believe I let it get this bad. A few days ago I was starting to feel off. I was really anxious, which is rare because I usually don't experience anxiety. It's usually just depression.

Just!

Anyway, I got a new puppy a week ago and I think he is making me feel anxious because it's like taking care of a baby since he is still only a month old. But that's not all. I went to my grandma's house last Sunday, and I was already feeling off, as my mind was somewhere else. I played with my cousins, but I felt disconnected the whole time. When I got home, I went for a walk with Oliver (my puppy) and my mom. We drove to this park and got into a stupid argument—I don't remember what it was about—and she got angry and left Oliver and me and drove home. I tried to walk him but this puppy is on crack or something. He was hopping around like a bunny rabbit, and got loose from his harness. It wasn't far, but I was getting itchy to death as we walked home.

That's when my anger and depression came fueling up. My skin was itching like crazy, which happens a lot because I am allergic to every fucking medicine and I can never just take a pill and feel better. I felt like I was going to drop dead carrying this jumping rabbit of a dog.

When we got home I went straight to my room, where the lid blew off. My mom was out walking and my sister and dad were outside.

My anger was rising and rising.

I Googled "least painful ways to die" and YouTubed it. I found a pretty dark video showing an overdose, running a car in a closed space, letting the gas fumes suffocate and kill you. I was about to jump out of my skin so I went downstairs to my medicine box. I got a bottle of Klonopin and lined up nine pills on the counter, crying my eyes out the whole time. I tried to wait for my mom's car to pull in the driveway, but she wasn't coming.

I couldn't scream or talk at all.

All I could think about doing was staring at the pills.

I poured a glass of water. Still no sign of my mom's car and my sister and dad were just chilling outside.

I was being held prisoner by my own depression.

My thoughts were getting so loud, like I was being yelled at to get out of the way of an oncoming train.

Then everything became silent. I grabbed the pills and swallowed them all down with water as quickly as I could. I went up to my room and laid on my bed, hoping the effects of the Klonopin would put me to sleep.

But then, as usual, I became a weakling and when my sister came up the stairs I yelled to her, "Take me to the ER!"

I got changed and packed a bag because wherever I was going I knew it was going to be for at least a couple of days. I sat on the couch while Alisa got my dad and told him what was happening with me.

I can't believe him. He has some nerve what he said to me.

"Nicole! Why would you do that? We just got you a new dog."

Like I chose to do this all out of my own free will?

"Dad, all I want to do is die! I can't take it anymore. All I want to do is escape this pain!"

What a stupid-ass to make that comment to me.

That's what I was thinking, kind of, even though it was my dad, who doesn't know what to do anymore and I can't blame him, but I guess he can't understand what I am going through, but still, I wanted to punch him in the face right then and there, even though I love him.

I went to Mather Hospital—again—in Port Jefferson. I knew it wasn't the greatest place, and I hadn't been there for a while, but man, that place went downhill! The psych emergency room was the biggest dump I had ever been to. I didn't remember it smelling this bad.

The room they put me in looked like a cage. It smelled like human feces, and there was a small hard couch I couldn't even fit on. There was no ventilation. No doctor or social worker came to evaluate me for the first three hours, and I felt like I was being held captive.

I would have rather died than gone there if I knew it was going to be that bad.

Another person was banging on the walls, screaming, so they had to be restrained and that frightened me and I started crying my eyes out.

That place was pure hell.

My mom and dad were beyond angry because of this environment. This beast across the room from me kept screaming bloody murder. I lost track of how many times he had to be put in restraints. I thought I was in a prison, with at least 10 bodyguards outside my door.

Five hours later, I was asking for a bed to sleep because I could not sleep on this cheap, tiny couch that was breaking my back. All I wanted was a gurney to sleep on. Everybody else had one!

Finally, at nine p.m., six hours after I arrived, I got a gurney and it was so refreshing to lie down, even though the pillow and sheets smelled like pee.

Still no social worker or doctor to see me or tell me anything.

Now I could understand why that guy lost his marbles. All he wanted to do was talk to a social worker—we all did. My mom made so many complaints to the hospital about how they were treating me—or not treating me.

Whatever . . . they suck.

On Monday, my mom took off from work and called our health insurance to complain about Mather. I had been there for a full day and still hadn't received any treatment—nothing. They didn't have any beds on the psych unit so until then I had to remain in this dump of a hallway in the middle of a really messed up scene, like a bad TV show.

Only this is real, and it's my life.

July 12, 2016

I was transferred to South Oaks Hospital in Amityville, where thankfully my aunt worked, so I knew I would be in good hands. There were no other beds available on Long Island, which just shows how broken the mental health system is out here. It's awful for people like me, or individuals dealing with substance abuse. Not that I have a substance abuse problem, but treatment for it is very scarce on Long Island and expensive.

South Oaks may be the nicest hospital I've been to. In the morning, my aunt visits me and brings me muffins!

I no longer feel suicidal.

All I want to do is go home, back to my new puppy, back to my job, if its still there.

I am going to beat this.

I am always thinking this, too, whenever things go off. I always do. I'm a fighter. All I need is medicine adjustments and I'll be fine.

I wanna go home.

I'm upset that I let it get this bad. I don't want this to be in this endless cycle. Like 10 years from now, if I have a family of my own, I don't want the same thing to happen so that Daddy has to explain to the kids that Mommy is in the hospital-again.

I will not be having children in the future.

I just decided that, after thinking it over, and whoa, that feels good. What a big weight off my chest. I would be so embarrassed if that ever happened so I just can't take that chance.

I'm no longer crying, which is good!

I feel like I'm in *One Flew Over the Coo Coos Nest.*

Everybody here is nice. There are normal depressives, but not everybody is depressed. Some have substance and alcohol abuse problems, but no one has to be taken down and everybody is nice to each other. We have Netflix! We're a nice mix of people struggling with all kinds of problems and no one is jumping out the window.

I'm kidding of course! Humor gets me through difficult situation. My roommate isn't crazy, which is nice, and she's normal and nice to me. She's the same age.

I just spoke to my doctor and it doesn't seem like I will be here past the weekend. He asked me if anybody in my family has a history of mental illness. I said my grandpa on my dad's side has depression.

"Your grandpa?" he said, like this was big news.

"Yup."

Thanks. Grandpa!

"Can you relate to him?"

I looked at the doctor and smirked.

That was a stupid question.

I was thinking that to myself, like what could I say?

"I guess so! He's my grandpa."

Why are we blaming this on somebody else? Can we really do that? If that's true, then who made Grandpa Nagy all depressed, and did he have a tumor, too? I don't think so.

All I want to do is go home. This shouldn't be happening to a normal girl like me. I didn't ask for this. I should be enjoying summer, getting sunburned, making money, and feeling tired for good reasons.

I just finished an intense semester at Stony Brook I deserve a break! But unfortunately, depression latches on to innocent people, sick or not. It's like a dark cloud that comes over you, and it's difficult to escape its shadow. You can pray all you want but it takes more than that.

I pray every night to God for me to get better, but like when I was standing over those nine pills in the kitchen I knew he didn't have that power. But I still feel God has me here for a reason and that's why I haven't died yet. I go to church and push myself through school and life because somewhere deep down inside me, through rough times, I know I have such a bright future ahead of me and I don't want to fuck it up.

All I wanna do is cry right now. I wanna go home.

I'm trying not to lose my mind. If I do, they won't let me go home.

Like my old therapist said, "You have to fake it till you make it."

That's not to say I am pretending to feel better, like some epiphany just came over me and I am all cured, but I have to fake my emotions in order to pull myself out of my room.

I received some insider training by other people here who said that if I participate in all of the therapies I will most likely get a reduced sentence.

Ha ha. That is a joke—the reduced sentence. Get it?

I find this technique helpful because I realize that when I do push myself out of my room into the different therapy groups I feel a lot better.

I haven't heard from Dr. Iyer since I've been here. It's not like I'm waiting to receive a call from her but it would have been nice to hear what she is doing, trying to work with the other doctors to get me out of here. I really want to go back to work as much as I can before school starts. I need money because I have a car payment and a dog to take care of and I don't even know how much my books are going to cost for fall semester.

I don't want Sergio to visit me. In fact, I don't even want him to know I am here. But before I tried to OD I texted him "I'm sorry" and my sister Alisa told him later what happened. Sergio has been with me so long and he knows everything I have gone through and he has always been by my side. I feel sorry for him sometimes because when I'm home and in a depression episode I just want to be alone. Sergio feels helpless. I feel bad sometimes, but I don't want him to think that he would never be enough for me.

God forbid I have to choose between life and death.

It's just my chemistry, so once in a while I go through this. Sergio will always be enough for me. He makes me so happy, and I love him with all my heart. This might sound like a cliché but here goes.

Sergio makes me feel like a princess.

I think that a lot. He is the most kind, genuine, and loving person I've ever met, and I could talk about him for hours.

If I were Sergio I would be not embarrassed, but I guess I would be tired because in his position he has to watch me in this battle I keep fighting, but eventually I end up on top because I am a fighter! I am sure by this point that Sergio does not care about being embarrassed because I have these issues because he's been there for me in similar situations a lot. But still, I don't understand how he can keep up with me, I mean seriously, I'm either not affectionate or I'm all fine and lovey-dovey.

He says I never want to spend alone time with him with intimacy. That's because of my medication and my chemical imbalance. My medicines make me less in the mood and sometimes I just don't want to be touched. I sound like somebody on a bad TV show, but it's how I feel because these medicines, they make you feel weird, like somebody else, maybe, whoever that might be.

Sometimes, Sergio blames me for everything and it makes me aggravated and depressed. I can't control how my meds make me feel. Sometimes I'm good and I'm like, "Let's do this, I'm ready, I got this." But not always, that's for sure.

If he can't accept that, I don't know if we're going to make it. He didn't blame me or isn't upset I'm here right now. As far as I know, when I'm in these places he is very supportive.

My parents just came to see me. They didn't bring anything I asked for—sweatshirt, T-shirts—didn't get it.

My mom is so good to me. I love my family. I don't know what I'd do without them. I feel bad when they bring me new clothes for when I stay at hospitals. I always end up getting random clothes. I ask for simple things from home, but I guess they can never locate the stuff I describe to them so they give up and get me new stuff. I appreciate it, but I don't want them to spend more money on me.

I want my favorite sweatshirt.

July 14, 2016

It's Day 5 inside this hospital. I'm getting into a daily routine. I pretty much know everybody's name, so I'm in with the crowd. I'm not a "newbie" anymore. I still haven't heard from Dr. Iyer and I don't know if the doctor here got in touch with her. My mom is coming at lunchtime to speak to him. I'm hoping I can get out by tomorrow.

I wanna be in my own home!

I know this time it was a really close call (technically) because I took all those pills but I didn't black out or die. I just got sleepy. Anyway, I feel better. I keep telling myself that the next time I'm this bad I'm going to just go to somebody and motion for help. This is because I truly want to get better and back to a normal life.

I don't want to be one of those kids that are in and out of hospitals, and become known to the staff as a regular. Being a regular is what Starbucks and Dunkin

Donuts are for.

God forbid, the next time this happens again the rest of my family will find out.

My dad's side of the family are like the majestic horses. They seem to have no problems or they are good at hiding them. It's like, "Don't ask. Don't tell." My grandpa on my dad's side has depression, but it must be well controlled because I never heard about it. My mom's side of the family is like *Everybody Loves Raymond* because everybody knows what's going on with each other and they are laid back and funny.

I love all of my family so that is just me ranting on.

I'm going home tomorrow!

Mom spoke to the doctor here and Dr. Iyer is going to adjust my medicine. I gotta make sure they give me something good tonight so I can sleep! I'm not going to tell anybody here that I'm leaving because I'd feel bad, like I was ditching them. I'll just wait till the morning.

I miss the sound of my iPhone ringing to wake me up. I'm not sure what I'm going to do first when I get home—probably take a shower, then play with Oliver, and call my job and tell them I'm alive. If anybody asks, I'm going to say I was having some tests done from my post brain surgery. Alisa told my cousin I was in the hospital but I don't know if she told her why.

I just ate dinner, which was pretty good. It was my

favorite meal—Penne el vodka, spinach, and rice pudding. We watched *Silver Linings Playbook*, which I suggested, because let's face it, I'm sure we all can relate to this, being in a psych hospital.

We went out to the courtyard and I was teaching yoga to another kid. He really enjoyed it and thanked me, and then another person jumped in.

I had an epiphany.

I was thinking that I should work here as a counselor. I could totally see myself working here in the future as a social worker! I really like it here, but enough is enough as a patient, having to put up with morning breakfast TV reruns of *Saved By the Bell*.

I haven't spoken to Sergio since Sunday. I didn't have a phone and I don't have his number memorized.

I'm a bad girlfriend.

July 15, 2016

Today I will be a free woman! I leave at lunchtime!

I didn't get too much sleep because of the excitement. Once I get home I need to shave because I'm starting to feel like a wooly mammoth, but at least I am wearing sweatpants. I won't even bother eating lunch because I know I will be spoiled with real food once I arrive home. I feel bad for the other members because I have gotten to know most of them, but I know they are in good hands. Eventually they will go home, too.

Once I get home I'll have to readjust myself back into my natural habitat. It will feel weird to nestle in my own bed, and I know I will be waiting for somebody to come alert me for group therapy, or I will be expecting loud noises from the TV room, or somebody will be crying and I will have to drown it out with my TV to sleep.

So what do I do with all this quiet and peace?

August 1, 2016

I got my job back at the special needs school in Smithtown. I really enjoy it, especially during the summer because I do not have to do as much work. There are less goals to reach with the students because it's summer school and it gives me a chance to relax.

I had to find a new therapist because Nikki moved. I went through two since I got home before I found my current therapist. The first one seemed a little senile because when I told her where I worked she said, "Oh, I have a grandson with special needs. Let me show you a picture of him," and for about 20 minutes she brought out photo albums, saying. "He's so handsome, isn't he?"

What if I was suicidal?

I was thinking that.

What if I were suicidal and this lady, who is supposed to be helping me, is blabbing on about her grandson and I can't get a word in?

I was definitely thinking that the whole time. She wasn't much help so I never went back.

The next therapist was located in Dr. Johnson's old office building. He's the perv doctor, so that location shouldn't have been an option in the first place but my mom insisted.

"Oh you'll never see him," she said. "Go for yourself, Nicole, and don't let that idiot sick guy prevent you from getting help."

She went on and on like that, so I did. Feeling anxious like shit.

As I walked in and headed down the hallway, guess who is on his way out? The doctor himself, yeah, it was him. I stopped dead in my tracks, like a deer in a headlight, and we met eyes, and I did a 180 and headed out the door. I jumped in my mom's car, crying my eyes out, having a full-on panic attack.

It's not like he would have even recognized me after a few years and be crazy enough to talk to me and say anything stupid, but maybe, who knows?

"What's wrong?"

My mom didn't put it all together until he came out of the building and then she looked at him and understood right away.

"I saw him!"

I was mumbling between sobs because this hit me so

fast I didn't even have time to think about not crying or letting that bastard upset me.

"He just came down the hallway, and I'm never coming here again."

I had nothing else to say.

It's not like this doctor raped me or anything like that, but I felt violated anyway because he reminded me of a time when I was in a really dark place and he didn't make me feel better. In fact, he made me feel worse—way worse.

In a way, I thought it was my mom's fault because she kept insisting I go because I probably won't see him and then this happened. I wanted to say, "Told you so!" but how did she know I was going to run into him like that and she is right that I need to see somebody and these therapist do not grow on trees even though some of them deserve to fall out of one.

After that, I went back. I was prepared this time and wasn't going to let anybody get in my way of receiving help. Unfortunately, or fortunately, depending on how you look at it, the therapist there at that same place didn't make the cut in my book. She just nodded and said okay to everything I said.

Really? So taking nine pills is okay and I should just go about my business?

Eventually, I found Stacy, who became my current

therapist through my school's counseling center. She is really good. She's different than any therapist I had before. If she wants answers—she get them. There is a saying, like "You can't beat the answers out of a dead horse," or something like that. During my bouts of depression I am the horse and she gets answers out of me without me even thinking.

She would be a perfect interrogator for the CIA. If a horse was her client and she needed answers, she would be able to get the information. She pushed me right away to dig down into myself, to seek answers and nobody has ever done that before. I hope she doesn't leave me one day because she's really good.

I always get anxious right before starting up again at school, and I always seem to make it through with a few depression cycles, of course, but maybe this time it will be better.

I have stayed involved with many of my volunteer activities and picked up a second job. I am into soccer again, even though my soccer career is technically over. I can still coach. For the last month, I have coached soccer two days a week and worked at the school, making good money and then spending it all, which has left me with nothing, but it is what it is.

Whatever.

I earned, and I've blown it.

I set up my field placement for the fall semester at Stony Brook, which I am really excited about! I am ready to get out and start helping people, making a difference and all that good stuff. I have to intern twice a week, and on top of that go to school twice a week, so I cut down my work to once a week. I honestly am not sure how I am going to do al of this but luckily I have Stacy to help me out.

August 28, 2016

First day of school was fine! I felt like a pro getting on the bus, excited for the new semester and all the projects and drama that come with it.

It's my senior year, which is not like senior year of high school where you could BS the your way through it. Compared to college, at least here, high school was a party. This year might actually be the roughest because the expectations are higher. There will probably be less reading, but way more writing. I know I will have to write a lot of papers and step up my writing.

Thank goodness I have a writing tutor!

As much as I'd like to say that this last year will be easy, and I'm familiar with everything so it should be cool, I know that's not really the case and I am just hoping that I can make it through this last year without any hospitalizations or getting sick.

My goal is clear.

I will be thinking this all the way through. So while other students are striving to get good grades, I will be striving to stay out of a psych ward!

Oh wow, my grades suck, but I'm not eating a bucket of meds for breakfast.

I mean, I'm going to try my best, but I'm not looking for any A's because B's are good enough for me and my parents are cool as long as I pass. On top of that, I will be learning much more though my internship. That's the one good thing about going to school for social work. I'm able to learn more quickly by *doing* social work instead of just studying about it. Obviously, the school part is just as important, but I feel so much better when I am doing something.

I need action!

November 2016

My internship hasn't been exactly what I thought it was going to be. For the first couple of months, I really resented it and felt useless, and I dreaded going. I have to complete a certain amount of hours in order to graduate—14 hours a week, so my plan was go in for seven hours, twice a week. However, the placement I had was in an after-school program for two hours and forty-five minutes, which obviously would not meet the time requirements. That meant I would go into the program office at like noon on Tuesdays and eleven o'clock on Fridays. My task manager wouldn't usually show up until like 1:30 p.m. I'd sit there for hours, bored out of my mind, doing absolutely nothing.

What did I do?

I took advantage of the situation, which is a coincidence because Advantage is the name of the program. I would just go there early and do my homework on my computer. This went on for months. I co-facilitated a group called "Girl Talk," which started out as a group just for girls (duh) intended to talk about issues going in a female student's life. It later turned into "Real Talk" because a lot of male students wanted to join in, but I think they just wanted to hang out there because they had crushes on the staff member I worked with.

I was still new, so for the first month or so I had to build rapport with them so they would respect me and treat me better. I tried to plan ahead for the group with activities and group discussions, but most of the time it just turned into a yelling match with the students and me and the staff member. The students were incredibly disrespectful and they just used the club as a place to hang out.

You want some "Real Talk?" Okay, you guys are awful!

I was thinking that much of the time, especially with some of the boys. Maybe they were doing this program for the wrong reasons—so that's their loss, not mine.

I talked to my supervisor at the agency about the issues that went on. He was really helpful and assisted me in trying to find work outside the program. I did everything right. I talked to my field liaison, but she wasn't much help and I honestly felt completely let down, like I failed the students and was going to be a horrible social worker.

I wanted to blame myself more than them.

I knew I couldn't start doing that, because that would be a deep hole to get out of, so I tried to fight myself on that one.

On top of that, the assignments just kept piling on. It's not like they were even hard assignments, but they were busy work and it was annoying. I kept pushing and pushing and remained positive at my internship. I developed lesson plans and instead of me presenting them I had the students do that so they would get involved. The more I did that, the more I realized they appreciated me. I continued working through school like an animal and involved myself in volunteer opportunities and got started on grad school things.

There wasn't enough work for me with my internship. I had to create it. I tried to work with the actual social workers in the school, but that didn't work out. I offered myself up to anybody. I would have done anything, like run errands for the social workers. I could understand that after six or seven hours of school the students didn't want to be tortured by more school so I switched to making fun activities. I bought materials to make stress balls or decorate mason jars, trying to create stress-relieving activities, because I couldn't do worksheets.

There were certain topics I had to abstain from while interning, too, like suicide, depression, and family issues.

But I always remained positive because I was representing my school, the agency, and myself.

I persevere, which is a new word I learned somewhere.

February 2017

I made it through another semester, and now, just a few months till graduation. Over winter break, I took another intersession course, worked at school, coached, and did grad school applications. It sounds like a lot, but I managed.

I still feel like a babysitter at the internship. It's not the most terrible thing in the world, but it's definitely not the social work experience I thought I'd be getting. Then again, everybody's first internship probably isn't life changing.

Am I really suited to become a social worker?

I keep thinking this because I don't like feeling uneasy for so long, which I have been doing because I assumed this profession is what I am destined to do but this experience is making we wonder if I'm right.

I have to remain positive.

I am trying to engage the female students into

conversations, and I've come up with lesson plans about mindfulness and stress.

Maybe I can take my own class because I can always get better with that stuff.

I advocated for more work within the agency and guess what? Ask and you shall receive. I started working on a project within the agency called ESG, short for the Emergency Service Grant. It's for individuals at risk of becoming homeless or are behind on their rent. People have to meet certain guidelines, like income, and the catch of this program is, a person has to show proof that going forward they can sustain on their own. I make phone calls to people who inquire about the services and ask them various questions to see if they meet the requirements, like if they have exhausted all of their means and this and that. I enjoy it because I am confident in my speaking, so when I was practicing with another intern she always suggested I take the lead.

I have good speaking skills by now and have learned to be good with people.

But the job is far away so I went back to my old internship with the mindset that I'll keep thinking positive and make plans to do things with the students, whether they like it or not. Sometimes I go to different groups where I know the students will take to me. I even went out of my way to talk with many of the female students and start simple conversations with them. I brought nail polish and offered to do some of the girls' nails.

Eventually a few of the female students fell in love with me and I spend the whole time taking to them and giving them advice. This is the only thing I look forward to because I feel like I am doing some good.

February 14, 2017

This is a sixth Valentine's Day with Sergio. He continues to work odd jobs—well not really odd, but low-end kind of jobs. He has his bachelor's in criminal justice but that really isn't enough.

I wish I could tell him that.

I think I should, but then I think I shouldn't, so I don't.

All the jobs he keeps applying for only required a bachelor's, which I guess he assumed should be enough. But the key word is *experience*. Nobody is going to hire someone with a degree without a least a minimum of three to five years of experience.

I feel bad for him because he is so intelligent, but he doesn't have the means to get his master's in something. I would never tell Sergio this, but it's frustrating because I know it's true and I wish things could be different for him so he could do what he really wants.

If Sergio can't find a real job or go on to get his master's degree then I can't marry him.

This is my belief that I think I have to hold myself to.

I don't know if that is shallow or not, but I have to be smart. I know what I want and my profession might not make me a lot of money, but I'm okay with that because my job is so rewarding, or at least I think it will be, and I better be right.

On the other hand, I will have benefits and healthcare.

Whoa, I sound like my mom.

I'm not sure if that's a good thing—sounding like my mom—but its true! Things aren't cheap on Long Island and I believe Sergio is the person I want to spend the rest of my life with so I hope all this career stuff can work out so we can do that.

He can't spend the rest of his life working as a mechanic or a waiter. Sergio is an intelligent person and I'd hate for him to not be able to do anything more like he can do. He always explains to me he has bills to pay and I understand that he pays for his own school and car, and has to pay for rent, too, which I still don't understand.

His step-dad is a dirt bag.

Can I say that? I just did, and I'm thinking it, but I'm not sure if it's okay to say it. I'm gonna stop now before I insult somebody, because that is not my intention.

I am proud of Sergio. He got his citizenship, which

is not an easy thing to do, and his bachelor's degree, even though it's a degree where you need another one to get a good job. I just wish he would apply himself more because he's so freaking smart and driven. Maybe he needs to take chances, but maybe he can't because he has to support himself.

I think there is some stigma brought on by our society, that you need to go to college and be successful in order to be happy. Sometimes I feel like I have to hold myself to somebody else's standards. I think Sergio feels it, too.

We have to figure this out.

March 2017

I went up to Albany again, this time with the School of Social Welfare. I wrote a letter to my Assemblyman beforehand and he emailed me back, saying I could meet him, and I did!

The State Capitol building in Albany is like a castle, like Hogwarts. I waited outside the chambers and went up to the guard and asked him to give a note to Assemblyman Alfred Graf, saying I have a meeting. I tried to sound professional and showed him the email and he was like "Okay, that's proof!" I wasn't sure it was going to work, but I did. He started walking to the door, and my friends were like "Ah, now you gotta talk, so what are you going to say?"

Ha ha, really funny.

But really, that's what I was thinking, that I better sound good when the Assemblyman comes out, which he did pretty fast.

Then, like usual, my public speaking skills kicked in and I introduced myself and we all spoke to him. The legislation we were lobbying on was called "Raise the Age." New York and I think North Carolina are the only two states in the U.S. that charge 16 and 17 year olds at adults. A lot of people, including myself, think that this is detrimental to young people.

Anyway, my assemblyman was not in favor of this. He was very quick to cut off one of my friends when he tried to explain his view. He basically shut us down and didn't really listen to us.

Assemblyman Alfred Graf didn't listen to us.

I was thinking, what a jerk, but then I thought about it some more and really appreciated this bad experience because not everybody I work with in the future is going to agree with me or my friends, but I have to give people an opportunity to explain their side.

Assemblyman Alfred Graf can learn that, too, one day.

Before we went to our legislative meetings we went to a rally outside and News 12 from Long Island interviewed me! My friend, Albert, was there, and he is so funny. I pointed out Doug Geed, the news guy, to Albert, and then I went to talk to Mr. Geed and asked for a picture. One thing led to another and he was so friendly and asked if he could speak to me! They put me in front of a camera and he was literally interviewing me!

He was interviewing *me*!

I couldn't believe it! I was kind of ↳

so I knew what I wanted to say in my head but ⌐

come out that way. Luckily, News 12 only shows small

clips of people speaking like I did so they used one of

the important points of my interview and it was on TV!

You gotta love News 12 because all they do is repeat

the same news all day. So anybody who watches it

probably saw me, maybe over and over.

The next day, I was about to do errands and I stopped.

I have to put on makeup because what if people recognize me and I look ugly?

I was saying that in my head, I admit it, because

thinking I could be surrounded while I was doing errands

and had to look good when I got stopped by people, and

say over and over, "Yes, I am that girl, thank you." This

short blast of possible fame was getting to my head and

making me delusional.

Pull yourself together!

That's what I had to keep telling myself. The thing is,

I never had an experience like this and I thought I was

famous and was letting this one moment get to my head.

I should never become a celebrity because I feel like I

could become an airhead.

The next day I went to work and a few people said

they saw me and I tried to seem nonchalant about it. I

dn't want my recent fame to make me seem arrogant.

Oh, my gosh, I am doing it now!

I looked in the mirror and had a little therapy session with myself.

Pull your crap together lady because you're not famous and you're nobody!

I had no trouble telling myself that because I was thinking it and just had to believe it, and I better do it before it's too late

April 1, 2017

News 12 just gave me my own show!

Ha ha if you fell for that—April Fools!

The real accomplishment will be graduating and getting into the Master's program at Stony Brook. I only have a month left of school and there is so much work to do with my thesis paper and all the busy work.

I really wish I had friends.

Okay, I have friends in class, but it's not like we hang out or anything.

I daydream about my pretend friends and me and about stuff we could do.

This may seem completely crazy, but it makes me feel better. I have these fantasies, but not in a weird way. Sometimes, I feel like a loner because I desperately want to have friends to talk to or to hang out and do things.

I have Sergio, which is great, but I can't bring him everywhere as a safety net.

He's fun and everything, but I need a change. I'm in college and I feel like I should be having the time of my life but it hasn't really turned out that way. I wish I would have lived in a dorm but it's too expensive and I live 15 minutes from school so there's no point.

I'm also glad I didn't go away to college because I see so many people around town who I went to high school with that went away to college and now they're like 500 pounds. All they do is party and drink and come back looking like Tracy Turnblad's mother in *Hairspray*.

I have one really good friend, but she is always working or studying, which is understandable—like it is with me—but when she's free and I see on Instagram that she's going out with her other friends, I get jealous. I'm not expecting her to invite me to go wherever she goes because that's silly, but I just want people to hang out with to have conversations with and eat or whatever.

College is supposed to be a time for me to explore and meet new people.

Maybe something is wrong with me.

I take it like this when I am alone in my room on a Friday or Saturday night and all I have to look forward to playing computer games. I am not alone all the time, but its enough to make me feel depressed sometimes.

April 8, 2017

Let it be known that on this day at 4:53 p.m. I received an email from my school, saying I got accepted into Advanced Standing for the School of Social Welfare.

I just freaking exceeded all expectations in my life's journey.

At one point of my life, I never thought I'd make it to the age of 18, and then 19, and then 20, and then 21, and I didn't think I would make it through four years of college. No way.

When I opened up the email I couldn't contain my excitement. I had planned on freaking out my mom by having a quiet but soft tone in my voice when I told her.

I wanted to say it like this:

"Mom, I have to tell you something, okay? Please don't freak out."

I know this sounds completely crazy, but I almost wanted to give her the impression that I just found out I was pregnant, but it didn't go that way, which is probably good. Anyway, I was too excited to speak at all and I just started screaming.

"Mom, Mom, MOM!'"

I ran down the stairs with my phone and she was asking me if I was okay?

"Nicole, you're scaring me!"

I started laughing.

"I thought you were having a seizure!"

In my twisted mind, I was like, "Oh, this is even better. She was just thinking I'm sick, but really I was about to deliver her great news!

I showed her the email and she was so happy. My sister and dad were right alongside her and they were both so happy for me.

I can't think of any higher achievement for myself after everything I've been through.

The next few weeks of school were not too bad. I'm almost at the home stretch, with five weeks left. For the most part I will not have any finals, expect for one, but it's a take home. The rest are presentations, but I'm not worried because I can practically do them in my sleep.

April 20, 2017

I'm trying to get more involved with clubs at school. I want to meet more people my age that I can hang out with so I am not so dependent on Sergio. It's coming down to the end of the semester so it's obviously going to take more time for me to do this.

My mom says that once I graduate and get a full-time job this feeling of needing a change is not going to go away. I'm not sure why.

In the back of my head I keep hearing voices.

Okay, I'm not really hearing voices, so no one is running to the ER or anything, but this is a gut feeling I guess, something telling me to break up with Sergio, to break up with him, I just said that, and to do it now!

How come my mind is telling me this?

This is somebody I have been with for half of my life, not really, but sort of, in my heart, at least, it's like that. We met in high school, but that's six years I've been dating him, and I love him, so why all of a sudden is my mind doubting my relationship?

I think my mind is playing games on me.

I need to talk to somebody. I told my mom how I was feeling and she tried to rationalize it by saying, "Well, Nicole, you've been dating Sergio so long you're probably growing apart and maybe you need a change."

Yeah, yeah, I see your point.

That's what I was thinking while I listened to her, but why?

What kind of bull crap was this that I was buying into?

I was completely out of it if I was determined to break up with him, thinking that he was holding me back from something, and I needed to end it as soon as possible. I had no control. I called my therapist right away and even she was confused. She knew how I was feeling, though, which led to her first question.

"Do I love Sergio?"

I hesitated.

"Well . . ."

"Nope!"

That's what she said!

Why didn't I answer?

Yes, holy mother of everything that is pure in this world, my answer without her even finishing the sentence should have been "Yes!"

April 28, 2017

I think I am having a mid-life crisis.

A week later, I tried to explain to my therapist that Sergio is holding me back. From what, I have no freaking clue, but he is.

My mind is in the gutter.

It just keeps telling me that I need to break up with him and I will be better off if I do. My therapist knows from our past sessions that I long for a more exciting social life. Maybe I am using this as an excuse to break up with Sergio. However, Sergio shouldn't have even been part of it because even when it's just us, sitting on the couch, cuddling together, we make jokes and we're happy and we find simple things to do that are fun.

For some reason though, I still can't shake this idea of why I want to break up with him.

"Do you want to date other people?"

Stacy asked me that.

"Because that's what it sounds like."

"I guess so."

Oh man, I just said that out loud. Do I have to own that now?

"Then there's your answer," she said.

I was having an out of body experience and saw myself and wanted to punch myself in the face. I wanted to scream at myself.

Lady, are you crazy? Wake up! Wake the fuck up! You are going crazy!

I guess that was my answer.

I left my session, telling Stacy I was going to call Sergio and break up with him that day.

On my way home I was feeling so excited, but also looking down at myself.

You stupid idiot, I hope you know what you're doing.

I called him and told him to meet me at the park by his house. He was confused why, and thought something was wrong—yeah—things were about to be for him.

I met him outside his house and I started off right away.

"I don't know how to say this, but . . ." and then I practically told him everything I told my therapist.

He was pissed off. He couldn't understand my reasoning, and I couldn't either. I made no sense and I didn't even have a legitimate reason why I was breaking up with him.

You butthead! At least have a real reason why you are breaking up with him or you look like a real fool!

I was thinking this, but I was still stuck in like, this mission, or something, to break up with Sergio. I told him I still wanted to be friends and he just looked at me and put his hands around my head.

"I hope you find somebody who has the same amount of patience for you as I do. I've been so patient with you and all your bullshit. But I'm not going to give up on us."

"Okay."

That's all I said.

Okay.

I wasn't offended because I know he was just angry and he was just lashing out. He walked back into his house and I drove down the street and pulled into a parking lot.

Reality hit and my out of body experience ended. I felt like I just got punched in the stomach, like a part of my body was just cut off, except it was me who did the punching.

What the fuck did I just do?

That's what I was thinking, that I just made the biggest mistake of my life. I immediately called him, and surprisingly he picked up.

"What do you want, Nicole?"

I poured out all of my feelings right there about how confused I was and how lost.

April 29, 2017

Sergio and I didn't talk for a day. I just felt depressed, not suicidal, just depressed. I told my mom what I did and even she was shocked.

I woke up this morning and was surprised to see a text from him. It wasn't "Good morning love" but it was still a reminder that he wasn't giving up. I called him in the afternoon and we went to the park in Stony Brook.

Things were a little awkward at first when we met up but that's only because I made it that way. We talked things out for an hour and we were together again. I guess it doesn't count as a break up, not really, since it was only for a day and there was no reason for it.

Sergio is the love of my life.

I know that's cliché, but it's the truth.

That morning after I called it a quits I felt like I couldn't function because knowing that I didn't have him made me feel weak. Sergio makes me a stronger person and there is no one else in this world I would rather share this life with. He accepts me for the craziness I create, and the struggles I create—in a good way. He supports me in everything I do and treats me like an angel.

There was no way I was ever going to let him go.

I don't care what Sergio does with his life. I mean, I want him to be successful, but it doesn't matter to me any more, as long as Sergio keeps loving me the way he loves me now. If he does, I will always stick by his side.

I'm pretty sure I found my soulmate.

I think going through this it has made our relationship stronger. Not that I'd ever want this to happen again, because I was bat shit crazy, as my professor would say.

So that was that.

May 2017

I'm so happy that today is the last week of interning. I am sad to be leaving the students because staff people are always leaving them. I found out that the staff only gets paid ten dollars an hour and that's not anything. I make more than that working at the school in Smithtown!

I am leaving on good terms, though, so that makes me feel a lot better. Looking back, I think this internship benefited me in some ways because I ran my own groups.

I'm so close to graduating I feel high on life or something.

It's not in a religious way, but I'm so excited to have two more days of school. Waking up and realizing you have no essay to write, a process recording to write, or anything homework-related is better than ecstasy—the feeling is indescribable.

My social life has been getting kinda busy now, too, which is good. I am starting to go out more with people— mostly Sergio's friends. When I'm old and crusty, I'd like to look back at my 20s and say I actually did a lot of things and say I had fun.

My future is all set, at least for the short-term as a graduate in two weeks with my Bachelors Degree in Social Work and starting grad school in the fall at Stony Brook. Some people I have talked to have said, "Oh, that's really hard to get into the master's program" and they say, "My son, daughter, niece, blah blah, applied for psych at Stony Brook and didn't get in."

First of all, psychology and social work are two different things, and second of all, the psychology program is very competitive.

I'm freaking Nicole Nagy, so you better believe I intend on making it in this program!

May 19, 2017

Let it be known that at four p.m. today I graduated from Stony Brook University!

Nobody can tell me I didn't finish anything.

Nobody can tell me that I need to wait.

Nobody can tell me any BS like that.

I don't know why I'm not more excited to graduate today. I think it's because I am so burnt out from five years of college, between Dowling and Suffolk Community College and Stony Brook. My parents are really excited for me but I feel like they're obligated to be since they are my parents.

No—I'm kidding, but I think I'm not like super pumped because I feel like I am never satisfied with my work. Don't get me wrong. It's an accomplishment, but I don't know.

I'm not greedy, like I should be pushing myself more, but that's my spiel.

Sergio was there for me on my big day and he told me how proud he was of me. A couple of years from now we could get our own place and be successful together, and I'll try to make him dinner even though I don't know how to cook anything. It will be great!

When I got to school to get ready for the graduation, I regretted not taking a Klonopin. There were so many students there and it was hard to find people I knew inside the building. I eventually started to recognize some of my classmates, but everybody was in their own cliques.

I just wanted to hide somewhere where nobody could see me.

I was thinking, "Just call my name when you're ready."

This didn't happen though, because I had to wait around in the hallway. Everyone was taking selfies with their friends and I was being awkward. I wasn't friends with everybody in my class. I maybe talked to a few people, but they were off doing their own things.

This shouldn't have even mattered!

I knew that, that I was graduating, so why was I so consumed with having to be with everybody else? I didn't even like many of the people in my program.

In less than an hour, I will have the most important thing—a degree. I will be a few steps closer to positively affecting lives.

The ceremony didn't even start and I already wanted to go home.

Luckily, my professor saved me because she had to rally everyone together. It was time. The music started and I felt so uncomfortable.

"I would like to walk out to the *Rocky* music!"

Everybody laughed, and I felt at ease. For some reason, joking around during tense situations makes me feel better! The ceremony didn't last long. I didn't fall when I crossed the stage to get my paper degree. My professor said my last name right. I didn't feel satisfied, but I was happy that everybody else was happy for me.

This summer, I plan to make the most of it. I want to hang out with Sergio as much as possible. We're basically married and we see each other every other day, at least. We go to the gym together three times a week and go food shopping. We just don't live together. But I can't wait for it because he makes me so happy and nobody makes me laugh as much as he does.

I am also going to be interning at Long Wood Middle School, which I am excited about because it's going to be a life changer for me, but also for the students, too, because I hope I can impact them in a big way.

That's my mission: to help people who need it so they won't go through what I did, and if they do, they know they have somebody who understands and can help.

That's me.

And that's what I think with my creative mind.

One Last Thought

I believe everybody has a story to tell and this is my story.

I feel obligated to share mine. I think we as humans have an obligation to share our struggles with the world because at one point or another we are all dealing with similar circumstances. I believe that if people share their own personal testimony of dealing with mental illness, or any type of struggles, then the world will be smarter about this stuff and do a better job of fixing it.

I know that not everybody wants to share their life story with everyone, but I'm determined to do it because I am passionate about helping and inspiring people, which I hope I've done with this book.

I've grown over the years since I started writing it, and many things that I've dealt with have changed me for the better. I don't regret anything because I feel that even all the bad stuff has helped shape the person I am today. I don't know what set of obstacles are to come.

I'm 24 and I have accomplished a lot. All I know is right now—Master's Degree, here I come.

This is not the end of me. This is just the beginning,

Nicole's Timeline

October 21, 1993	Born in Smithtown, New York at St. Catherine's Hospital
September 1996	Preschool at Red Robin Country Day School
August 2008	Anxiety episodes begin
September 4, 2008	First day of high school
June 2009	Freshman year ends as anxiety grows
September 2009	Take bus to school for first time
October 2009	Anxiety episode in school leads to ER and psych center
June 2010	Family finally secures a house and my own room
August 2010	Begin working as assistant coach for girls' soccer team
September 2010	Meet Sergio, fall in love
February 2011	Meeting with Louis Medina from Suffolk County Youth Bureau
June 2011	Begin working at Suffolk County YouthBureau
February 2012	Accepted to Dowling College

June 2012	Graduation from high school
September 2012	Begin studies at Dowling College
December 2012	Withdraw from Dowling to deal with depression
January 22, 2013	Visit Mather Hospital ER for OCD and major depression
January 27, 2013	Mather outpatient clinic
January 29, 2013	Psych testing for unexplained episodes of paranoia and anxiety
March 2013	Seizures begin
April 29, 2013	Neurologist reviews MRI, which reveals brain tumor
May 2, 2013	Admitted to NYU Hospital
May 10, 2013	Brain surgery
May 13, 2013	Discharged to return home after surgery
June 2013	Try to reconcile reasons for anxiety and depression
June 2013	Write letter to Suffolk County Radiology, protesting treatment
August 13, 2013	Back in hospital because of possible seizure
August 27, 2013	Last day of work at bakery before school starts
February 2014	Headaches continue unchecked
July 2014	Last day working at high school
September 2014	Scholarship offer from Dowling
September 2014	Transfer from Dowling to Suffolk Community College
October 21, 2014	21!

February 2015	Struggle through college while adjusting to medications
August 2015	Back in hospital while trying to finish school
December 2015	Complete first semester at SUNY Stony Brook
February 2016	Working, going to school, trying to avoid more hospital time
July 12, 2016	Admitted to South Oaks Hospital
July 15, 2016	Released and sent home
August 28, 2016	First day of school
March 2017	Trip to Albany with School of Social Welfare
April 2017	Make best effort at school to expand social life
April 28, 2017	Break up with Sergio
April 30, 2017	Back with Sergio
May 2017	Graduate from Stony Brook with BA in Social Work
December 2017	Share my life story with the world

Acknowledgments

To my mom, dad, and sister—the best family in the world. Thank you for your constant support through all of the obstacles I faced and for never giving up on me.

Sergio—what can I say? You have stuck by my side since the day we met. These past seven years with you have been amazing and I can't see myself with anyone else. Thank you for sticking by my side during my darkest moments and for continuing to love me through all of them.

Jill Pozderec—thank you Aunt Jill! The design of this book exceeded all my expectations and I am grateful for your assistance taking on this huge project.

David Tabatsky—thank you for all the work you have done with this project. You have been very supportive of me and truly understand my mindset, and not once have you ever tried to change the originality of my words or who I am. I am forever in your debt.

Louis Medina—you are the most genuine person I have ever met. Thank you for taking a shy girl under your wing and exposing me to the great work that you do. Without you I probably would not be pursuing this educational path. You helped shape me into the woman I am today by inspiring me to find my voice, a voice that won't stop.

About the Author

Nicole Nagy is a graduate of SUNY Stony Brook and is currently studying for her Masters Degree in Social Work. She lives on Long Island.

Please Visit

www.acreativemind-tdotmi.com

You can reach Nicole at

acreativemind.tdotmi@gmail.com
www.acreativemind.tdotmi@gmail.com

CPSIA information can be obtained
at www.ICGtesting.com
Printed in the USA
BVOW06s1918061217
502130BV00021B/175/P